The Gift of Experience

EXCERPTS FROM CONVERSATIONS WITH 21 MEN WITH HEMOPHILIA AND THEIR CAREGIVERS

THIS PROJECT WAS SUPPORTED AND FINANCED
BY
THE BOSTON HEMOPHILIA CENTER

INTERVIEWS AND TEXT BY
LAURA GRAY
and
CHRISTINE CHAMBERLAIN

RESEARCH ASSISTANT
MICHAEL HOERMAN

BOOK DESIGN
CHARLES CHAMBERLAIN ~ CAMDEN WRITERS

Some comments on *The Gift of Experience*

"*The Gift of Experience* captures the lives and perspectives of people with hemophilia in ways that the American media has repeatedly failed to do. There is vitality in these personal stories of hemophilia and diverse perspectives on how to persevere under conditions that are man-made as well as a natural inheritance.

Laura Gray and Christine Chamberlain have done a tremendous job weaving these oral histories into a narrative that allows their subjects to speak for themselves. *The Gift of Experience* is a 'must read' for anyone interested in the illness and disability experiences of people with chronic diseases as well as those with bleeding disorders.

Stephen Pemberton
Historian and Author

"You provided what so many of our patients really need - a voice, and people who will actively listen. It is obviously very healing for the patients and their families, and for their providers, too.

Thank you again for this. It is really a gift."

Bill Theisen, RN
Division of Infectious Diseases
Brigham & Women's Hospital

"The stories have reawakened aspects of living with hemophilia that I had seemingly forgotten. This book is moving and inspiring, a hopeful account of the human experience."

Avida

"Thank you very much for doing the *The Gift of Experience* and for sending me a copy. I started reading it immediately. I like the idea of the book as it is an excellent memorial to the lost generation."

Carol K. Kasper, MD
Emerita Professor of Medicine,
University of Southern California

"The interview is like an intervention, the effects of which continue to be felt. I find myself talking more with my family and friends about the hemophilia experience. Their reactions have surprised me in good ways. I realize that my view of my experience has already been profoundly altered, not only by thinking about my own life, but especially by hearing about the experiences of others with this illness. To that insight, I now add the response of family and friends who are eager to learn more."

Dr. James Martinowsky

"Once I picked up *The Gift of Experience,* I was overcome with emotion, not just when I read the chapter on my father, but when I saw that there were other families who had had similar experiences to my own. For the first time in my life, ever, I was in the company of other women who could "get" how it felt to be the daughter of a hemophiliac."

Anne Drummey

Center for the History of Medicine
Francis A. Countway Library of Medicine
10 Shattuck Street
Boston, MA 02115

Fourth Edition

For additional copies of this book, contact:

The Boston Hemophilia Center
Mid Campus-3
75 Francis Street
Boston MA 02115-6110

Library of Congress Number:
ISBN: 978-0-9802405-2-8

Published for the Boston Hemophilia Center by
Camden Writers, Brunswick Maine 04011-1912

This book was printed in the United States Of America

CONTENTS

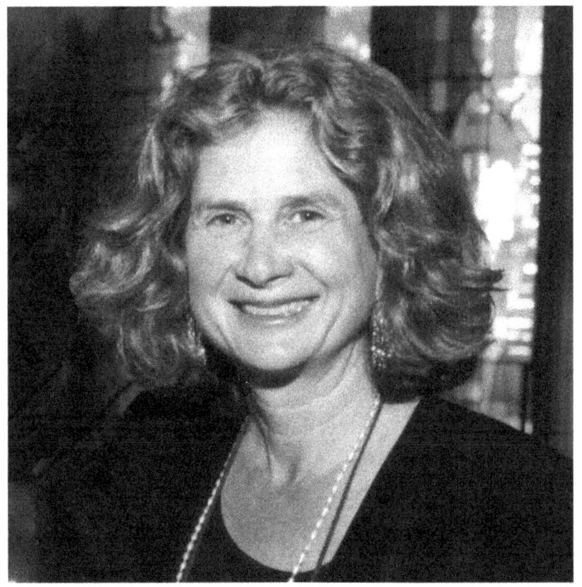

Laura Gray grew up in Newton, Massachusetts and graduated from Smith College School for Social Work in 1979. She has been at Children's Hospital for the past fifteen years and has been the social worker for the adult and pediatric patients at the Boston Hemophilia Center for the past ten years.

THE GIFT OF EXPERIENCE:

LAURA GRAY:

When I started my social work job at the Boston Hemophilia Center in the mid- 1990s, I knew nothing about hemophilia. I had never heard of factor or fresh frozen blood or cryoprecipitate. I remembered that the country's blood supply was unsafe in the latter 1960s and into the 1980s, but I had no idea what effect that had on people with hemophilia. I had never met a person with HIV and I knew very little about hepatitis C. I also didn't know that hemophilia was primarily a male disease and that it can be passed on through the generations. I didn't know any of this.

My job was to be a resource to these men and their families. I was supposed to understand the challenges of coping with this disease and offer support. While I had been a social worker for many years, I had no idea what the unique challenges or the particular needs of this community were. To be effective in my job, I needed to listen and learn.

Over the years, I was fortunate enough to get to know many of the men in our Center. I met them in the clinic or went to see them in the hospital if they had been admitted for care. I learned that there really was no effective treatment for hemophilia until the early 1970s. I also learned that there was a safety problem with the blood supply between the late '60s and the mid-'80s, when hepatitis C and HIV/AIDS were transmitted through the use of blood and blood products to thousands of men with hemophilia. The community was devastated. The more I listened, the more I learned and the more respect I developed for each and every one of these men. I learned about courage, perseverance, pride and resilience. I witnessed how love, humor and faith were essential ingredients to handling the pain, disappointments and devastating loss.

I want their stories to be told. I believe that what they have to say is critical not only for kids and families growing up with hemophilia today, but also for those who study the disease and want to better understand its effect on people's lives. This is also a book for anyone who wants some guidance and inspiration when facing his or her own difficult situations.

From 2004 to 2005 Christine Chamberlain and I conducted an oral history project called "The Gift of Experience." We interviewed 21 men with hemophilia A or B who are treated at the Boston Hemophilia Center. The book is a compilation of quotations from those interviews.

Also included are quotations from doctors, nurses and a social worker who have cared for people with hemophilia over the past forty years. The audio tapes and transcripts of the interviews are stored in the Center for the History of Medicine at Harvard Medical School's Countway Library in Cambridge, Massachusetts. This project was supported and financed by the Boston Hemophilia Center, a comprehensive treatment center based at Children's Hospital and the Brigham and Women's Hospital in Boston.

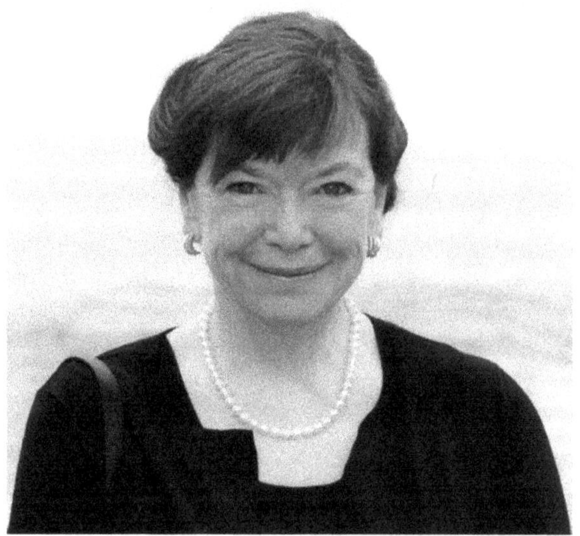

Christine Chamberlain is a principal partner of Camden Writers, a Maine-based company that produces memoirs and oral histories for individuals, families, family businesses and institutions.

Christine grew up in Cambridge, Massachusetts, was a history major at Wellesley College and has lived and worked for extended periods in the Middle East, the South Pacific and the United Kingdom.

CHRISTINE CHAMBERLAIN:

Our orientation to medicine — the belief that somehow, someone will pull an answer out of his or her bag of magic tricks — renders it counterintuitive to embrace the idea of a disease for which there is no treatment. Worse yet, our faith is severely threatened when we learn that the cure, at the least, infects and, at the worst, kills. Sadly, this is exactly what happened to the 17,000 men suffering from hemophilia prior to 1985, when the life-giving blood with which they were infused on a regular basis was found to be contaminated. Most of those men died. Those who did not, live under the Damocles sword of HIV and hepatitis C.

In the following conversations, we hear from individuals who shared the experience of hemophilia during a particularly difficult period. Even the most pedestrian procedure — having a tooth removed — required hospitalization. When they did go into the hospital, they often dealt with uninformed medical personnel and redundant bureaucratic procedures that made a difficult time almost untenable. Because the total population confronting hemophilia was relatively small, the level of understanding both inside and outside the medical community was low.

The development of clotting factor concentrates greatly enhanced the quality of life for men with hemophilia. Factor concentrates could be stored in a domestic refrigerator and administered quickly and in smaller volumes, providing much greater freedom for individuals. Home treatment became possible and lengthy hospital stays were greatly reduced. Unfortunately, this promising development was reversed when the nation's blood supply was found to have been contaminated with the HIV virus.

Through these stories we learn about the art of accommodation. How do you deal with constant pain or face the disappointment of standing on the sidelines when you want to be in the game? What eases the grief of losing friends and family members to HIV, and how do you compensate for the relationships you can't have and the jobs you don't get? Into what corner do you stuff the anger? What risk is worth taking and who decides?

The stories in this book are not easy ones, but they are, against all odds, an insightful testament to optimism and determination. The population is specific but the journey is universal. Any person facing grief or hardship would do well to enter these conversations, for herein he or she will find the essence of resilience from people who have run the expert trail.

It is fundamental to yearn to be accepted for who we are and to be treated with compassion, respect and understanding. Our hope is that reading these accounts will heighten awareness, not only of hemophilia, but also of any disease that profoundly affects the quality of life in those around us, and better equip us to nurture dignity, opportunity and hope wherever we can.

As one of our participants said, "This is not an overlay on my life; this is my life. I have had hemophilia since the day I was born. This is me."

EARLY HISTORY*

References to excessive and unexplained bleeding have been made since antiquity. In the Talmud, a collection of Jewish Rabbinical writings from the 2nd century AD, it was written that male babies did not have to be circumcised if two brothers had already died from the procedure. In the 12th century AD, an Arabian physician from Cordoba named Albucasis wrote of males in a particular village who had died of uncontrollable bleeding. Occasional references to bleeding can be found in the scientific literature of following centuries.

In the United States, the transmission of hemophilia from mothers to sons was first described in the early 19th century. In 1803, the Philadelphia physician Dr. John Conrad Otto wrote an account of "a hemorrhagic disposition existing in certain families." He recognized that a particular bleeding condition was hereditary and predominately affected males. He traced the disease back through three generations to a woman who had settled near Plymouth, New Hampshire, in 1720. The word "hemophilia" first appeared in a description of a bleeding disorder condition at the University of Zurich in 1828.

*Courtesy of the National Hemophilia Foundation, 2007

I never could distinguish between my experience in life as a human being as something different from my experience in life as a human being with hemophilia. I couldn't really imagine what it would be like to not have this. If you start to go down that road, then you can start to think a lot of things that are very painful and difficult. Maybe I just instinctively thought, "I can't go there."

Somehow, the key to living a joyful and happy life is not to wish that you were somebody else. I think the challenge that we face—that I faced and that everybody faces—is to live the life we've actually got and not to spend our time preoccupied with fantasies about lives that we could have lived.

Robert Massie

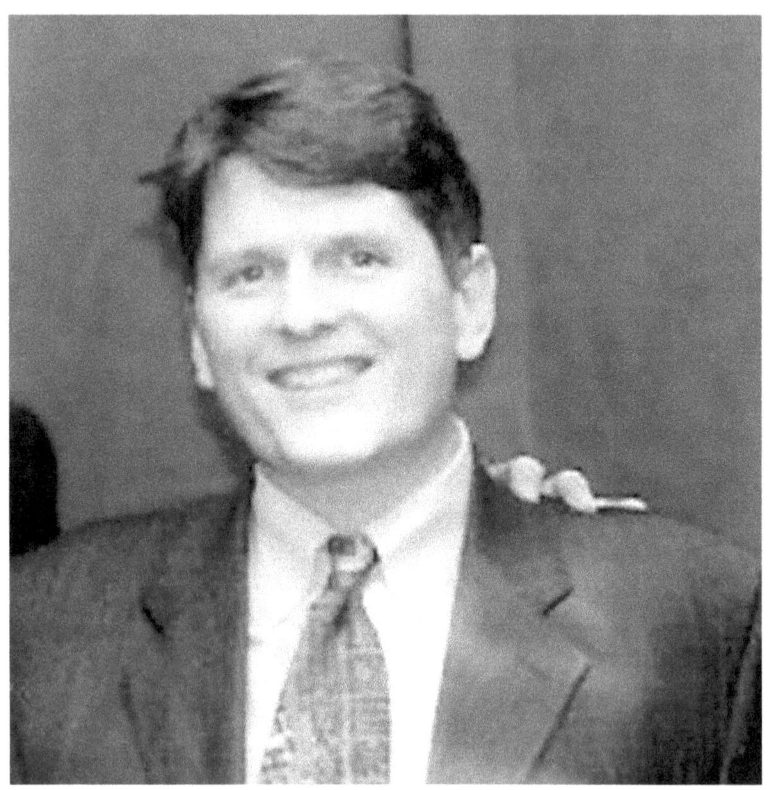

Robert Massie

ROBERT MASSIE

Mr. Robert Massie was born in 1956 in New York. His parents, both of whom are writers, produced a book, "Journey," documenting the family experience with hemophilia. Following college, Robert attended divinity school and was ordained as an Episcopal priest. He later received a degree from the Harvard Business School. Robert has three children and is profoundly concerned with issues of social and political justice. Robert is HIV positive and is waiting now for a liver transplant as a result of hepatitis C.

My uncle came over and was playing with me when I was about five months old. He'd been tossing me around, and after he left I had a couple of bruises. That struck my parents as odd. I think they then sought medical guidance on what this might be, and that led to a series of tests that eventually led to the diagnosis when I was about six months old. I would imagine that my experience is similar to others. Because it's something you're born with, there's no point at which you suddenly go, "Oh, my goodness! That's what I have!" It's just part of who you are and what happens as you achieve gradually deepening understanding of what it is.

When I look back on my childhood, I seem to have a rather selective memory, because what I remember are mostly very good things. I have lots of normal childhood memories of doing things with my parents or playing with my sister, watching television programs or going away in the summer. Those things are very, very vivid.

I didn't really start to have joint problems until I was about three or four. One quite vivid memory that, in retrospect, definitely takes on certain meaning, was in nursery school when I was four years old. I can remember being able to run, which is something I lost in the ensuing years.

I had a terrible bleeding in my left knee when I was about five that incapacitated me for many weeks. My leg bent up, as joints do, my muscle atrophied, and I was never really able to walk properly again. The only way they could get me walking was to put a brace on my leg. I wore a left leg brace from the time I was five until I was twelve.

I've kept two or three of the braces, partly because they were so much a part of my childhood. It just didn't feel right to throw them away. The slightly later ones were beautifully handmade structures, the work of a brace maker in New York. I walked like sticks, a stiff-legged person. That was the hard part of my childhood. I still feel sorrow, even though I don't really remember it, and what I feel sorrow about is the process of losing the ability to walk as a child. You go from being able to run to being in bed for a long period of time, then, when you get out of bed, you just can't walk again.

An important piece of this story is regaining the ability to walk later, when I was around twelve. Now I can walk and I've had two knee replacements. Even in the last six weeks, I've made a great advance, which is that I've been able to get back on a bicycle.

I used to ride my bicycle a little bit, but after the knee replacements I couldn't ride. My wife is a designer and an architect, and we were talking about what exactly it was that was keeping me from riding a bike. We realized that it was the length of the cranks that attached to the pedals, so I found an adjustable crank to make it shorter. Then I bought a recumbent bicycle so I was lower to the ground and didn't have to hop down. The recumbent actually has three wheels. It's a sort of tricycle, so I don't have to worry that much about being sure-footed on either leg. As a result, I've been able to do an incredible amount of bicycling in the last six to eight weeks.

I almost never go out without thinking what an incredible miracle it is that somebody who could not walk is now out there biking around on his two steel knees.

I think if you have hemophilia, or any chronic illness, or really any identifying feature that makes you different, you have to cope with the experience of presenting yourself to a new group of children or adults, in any setting. You have to negotiate the reaction that they have to you.

Having braces was disturbing to other children in the short term. In kindergarten and first and second grades, I was trying to fit in, and there were a lot of things I couldn't do. Leaving aside for a minute misunderstandings and anxieties that people had about hemophilia, there were certain sports I couldn't do. In second or third grade, during recess most boys ran out and played kickball or ran around and did stuff.

A lot of the girls played jacks. I couldn't go out and run around with the boys, but I was a boy so I couldn't really play jacks. Finally, I decided, "Screw that. I want to learn to play jacks." So I did and I became very good at it.

I ended up getting along very well.

One of the very deep traits I have developed in order to survive or flourish, is, in a sense, to convey reassurance to the person I meet. This is something inherited. I think I still do it and I think it's led to some interesting aspects of how I've lived my life. I'm used to conveying a sense of reassurance and confidence to people.

"Although I may have these problems, you don't have to worry about me; I'm okay. It's going to be all right and we can be friends."

I've lived my whole life as an activist — somebody who's been very interested in social justice issues, basic problems of fairness in our society, and I've asked myself many times why. I am a privileged white male from the Northeast whose parents went to good colleges on scholarships, yet I have this burning passion for making the world a better place.

I have this almost dual identity. Yes, I am a privileged white man, and yes, I grew up in this place where I was immediately categorized and judged on the basis of nothing that I had any control over, nothing that really mattered. I feel very deeply about issues like discrimination, exclusion, all of those issues, at a political level, a social level and a spiritual level, and I feel very deeply for people who've experienced them.

I think that sensitivity comes directly out of my experience as a child and knowing what it's like to be rejected, knowing what it's like to have to have enough self-confidence to reintroduce yourself repeatedly to a group, and then knowing that eventually one can win acceptance.

It's sad that human beings have this reflex to be scared of people who are different. I think that one of the things we have to learn as human beings — and one thing that I hope I've conveyed to my children as a parent — is that that reflex is something we have to train out of ourselves if we're going to live in a fair and peaceful world.

I have remained a very curious man. I'm interested in almost everything. For me, it's always been part of the same desire to know and understand the world, and that curiosity really drove a lot of things. I think my parents deserve great credit because their attitude was, "This is a very hard thing. You are faced with a tremendous challenge and we're going to help you as much as we can, but you need to keep in mind that you are a good person. You have tremendous value and whatever you run into is not going to ultimately stop who you become."

My parents didn't sugarcoat nor did they try and make everything work perfectly for me, but they gave me a tremendous boost of confidence.

When I was in bed for long periods of time, my parents were both very generous with their time and energy. Even when their own sense of what the future was going to be was uncertain, they presented me with a sense of hope, a sense of energy. They also really helped me feed the life of the mind.

We were living in this little house, and basically the only access I had to the outside world when I was in bed was television, books and whatever my parents could bring home. When I was 10, 11, 12 years old, I'd sometimes miss as many as a hundred days of school. I would read everything that arrived in the mail. If the *TV Guide* came, I'd read it cover to cover. I could have told you the price of any tent or any shotgun in the Sears Roebuck catalog, even though I didn't own either one of those items. I read magazines and I read whatever books I could pull off the walls.

I think my parents encouraged that as a way of saying, "You can bridge this gap."

When you live with hemophilia, you are constantly facing disappointment, and coping with disappointment is very hard as a child. It's a series of very hard blows and not everyone can survive them. To lose your ability to walk is terribly disappointing, but more frequently the problem is that you want to go on the school field trip on Friday.

Through Monday, Tuesday and Wednesday you hear all the kids getting prepared for that and you're excited. Then on Thursday you have an ankle bleeding or a knee bleeding and you can't go. They all go off on the school trip and then you hear about what a great trip it was when you get back to school the following Wednesday. Those kinds of experiences were very, very frequent, from as little as "Tomorrow morning I want to go outside and play in the leaves because it's autumn or out in the snow because it's winter."

Then you get up and you can't.

I never could distinguish between my experience in life as a human being as something different from my experience in life as a human being with hemophilia. I couldn't really imagine what it would be like not to have this. If you start to go down that road, then you can start to think a lot of things that are very painful and difficult. Maybe I just instinctively thought, "I can't go there."

Somehow, the key to living a joyful and happy life is not to wish that you were somebody else. I think the challenge that we face—that I faced and that everybody faces—is to live the life we've actually got and not to spend our time preoccupied with fantasies about lives that we could have lived.

Once you've made mistakes, once you've made choices in life, you can always go back and try to replay that tape and say, "Well, I wish..." Well, that's not productive either. I mean, there has to be some way to accept where you are and then move from that point. That's the way I dealt with it.

Now, that's not to say that it didn't hurt me. I mean, it did hurt me, these disappointments, particularly being such a gregarious child and being very interested in everything. So a chance to go out with friends and discover something new and have that cut short — very hard, and that happened many, many, many times.

We rehearsed and rehearsed and rehearsed for a nursery school play, and on the last day I had an ankle bleeding and I could not be in the play. I remember my father carrying me and sitting me next to the stage so that I could sing the songs with the other kids. And, you know, my heart ached. I wanted to be up there doing the things I'd learned to do and I couldn't.

The great challenge I have faced in the last two years is that having gone through all this and dealt with hemophilia and HIV, then being lucky enough to get an extraordinary job managing a national coalition of environmental groups and institutional investors, going to all kinds of places and really having an impact in ways that I could never have really imagined, I suddenly find that my hepatitis C has advanced so far that I have really serious liver cirrhosis.

I was supposed to give a set of speeches at a huge international gathering called "The World Summit on Sustainable Development" in Johannesburg. This was the culmination of several years of work and represented the coming together of many different pieces of my life. But I couldn't go. I couldn't go because I was still recovering from my knee surgery and we realized that one of the reasons I wasn't recovering very well was because I had such serious liver problems. I had to step down from my job.

I realized in one very painful period in January of 2003 that if I took any more steps to benefit this organization, it was a step against my health.

Letting go of my job, coming back and sitting here in Somerville and deciding that that part of my life was over — how do I make sense of that? But there are some happy sides to it. One is that people come to see me, which is very nice. I have also used the Internet the way I would have used it as a child, so it's like a sabbatical, which I had wanted. I just didn't want it in this form. That's just an example of this consistent challenge to me all the way through my life.

I think that everybody who goes through a hard experience, whether it's a medical experience or the experience of discrimination or unhappy family life, has to come to terms with, "All right, this is what's happened to me."

They have to say, "Because it's happened to me, I can't understand anybody else and they can't understand me. This is a unique set of experiences. I am the only one who has experienced it, and I've suffered in some unique way." That can become a very isolating experience, or it can become a kind of bridge. It can be a bridge from my unique set of experiences. My experience becomes a window into a lot of other people's experiences, and puts mine into context.

Nelson Mandela spent 10,000 days — 27 years — in prison. Nineteen years in the same cell. I'm sitting at home with fine foods and access to the Internet and no restrictions — no real restrictions on me of any significance. I guess that's what I mean. It allows me to bridge and say, "Well, yeah, certain things I'm going through are tough, but not really that tough." And this isn't just me sugarcoating, this is really an insight that allows me to experience a great deal. Once you've gone through the sorrow of a disappointment, you can find all kinds of new touchstones for joy and for peace, for inner calm and for being able to give, not just to be the recipient, but to actually give.

That all has its roots in the great love and generosity that I experienced as a child from the people around me.

I was in Amsterdam about eight or nine months ago and I visited Anne Frank's house. I saw the room where she sat and wrote every day for more than two years, and I thought about what it would be like to be a young girl under those unbelievably trying conditions, with the threat of death hanging around you at all moments. I thought about what it would be like trying to grow as a human being under those circumstances.

And I thought about the fact that I am living with people who care about me, in a comfortable house, with the ability to go anywhere. I was moved by that awareness, very deeply moved.

I understand on some level how people could reach a point where they feel so battered that they become victims, but I have a very deep sense that one should do everything possible in one's power to move back to a position of agency and action. If you get thrown into the experience of victim, it's a terrible thing. It is a paralyzing stance, one that allows you ultimately only misery and passiveness.

There are areas in my life where I had no control and where bad things, or sad or painful things happened to me, but what was key for me was to define and move forward in areas where I could grow and change and feel happy. That's a big part of who I am.

I don't condemn people who feel terribly burdened by what has happened to them. It's an understandable human response. But as long as people remain in that place, where they're focused on all that has been taken away from them, with this image in their head of the way life should have been as a source of pain and anger and frustration, I think they are putting themselves in a position where they can never be happy.

I understand how people find themselves in that place. I have certainly been there sometimes. But I think spiritual growth is about moving away from the pictures in our head about what we deserve, what we've earned, what we ought to have and what is fair, into what we actually have, what is happening right in front of us. There are all these things that we take for granted, that are unbelievable gifts — to start with, the ability to draw a breath and live.

Now, with the perspective of an adult, I can recognize that I went through many, many experiences of truly awful pain. I mean, not just discomfort, not just being in pain, but of real agony. I do block those things out to some degree. I can approach the hazy edges of the memory, but it's very hard for me to go back in. I think part of my mental equipment is that once I survived those things, I wanted to delete them.

I had many terrible joint bleedings and the pain of joint bleeding is like torture. Your joints become all the metaphors for terrible pain. It's like they are being broken in slow motion, like they're being burned. The pressure of a bleeding joint is particularly terrible because you have a sense of this massive, enormous force growing inside your joint.

I had bad reactions to pain medication. When I was given codeine, for example, it tended to intensify my pain. When I was a child, they were reluctant to give things that might be habit-forming, so there just weren't very many things available to me at that time.

In my case, the main treatment for pain was ice. The pressure of having any ice on a swollen knee was agonizing in itself. There were times when my knees hurt so much I couldn't bear the weight of a sheet. To put your bleeding ankle, inflamed and in terrible pain, into a bucket of ice is a hard thing to do. If you succeeded in keeping it there, it could numb the joint, but it intensified the pain to put it on the ice.

I feel lucky in the sense that these experiences didn't kill me or kill my mind, because I do have a strange recognition now that I did not have as a child that these were far more horrendous events than I recognized at the time. For me, it was just something you survived; you got through.

There's kind of a pattern for bleeding. The first part is this dawning recognition that something is wrong. It's very subtle at first. I used to call it having a "feeling." It's as though the joint was slightly — not tingly, but just that you had an unhealthy awareness of the joint. You'd be walking around and suddenly you'd find yourself thinking, "This knee, something is not quite right."

Then there'd be a period of the onset of pain and discomfort. One of the things that's critical about that period is going from a vague feeling to awareness: "I'm now entering into a problem." It's a very hard thing to recognize.

Then I'd have to alert my parents. They would have to call the doctor.

The doctor would have to come over. During that whole period, the pain would be getting worse and worse and worse, and if you were unlucky, the graph would go right through the roof. You would then be entering a crisis period where you'd think of running around a burning house trying to figure out whether there is any exit. For a long time, the answer would be no. Then whatever the period, however long it took — a few hours, a day, whatever it took — you'd come down and the crisis would be more or less over, sort of like coming over a mountain.

Now you're at this enormous long plateau and desert, which you have to cross because the knee or ankle or whatever could sometimes take weeks to go down. Here you were, doing all these activities, and then you have this bleeding. You have to come through it, then you have to readjust, then it can all happen again.

Sometimes it was an issue of pride.

I remember one occasion when I was very active and my father said, "Be careful."

And I said, "I'll be all right."

Then I had a bleeding and I didn't want to admit it because he'd been right. Once, and I'm sort of ashamed to say this, my knee started to bleed in the middle of the night after a very active, fun day. I woke up and I didn't want to tell my parents, so I strapped my leg into a brace and I went to school with a full bleeding, then waited about two hours until I could call my parents and tell them.

"Oh, oh, I have a bleeding knee."

It was a total farce! And my parents were not judgmental. They didn't say, "Oh, I told you so," or anything like that. But the deception was still in me, I didn't want to admit that there was a connection.

I have diaries from when I was eleven and twelve. I reread them recently and one of the heartbreaking things is that I'm so chipper in these writings.

"Oh, I've learned this and I did this today. And I'm really looking forward to going back to school."

Then the next entry is, "Well, I had an elbow bleeding, knee bleeding and couldn't go back to school." Then I filled several pages with, "Well, I did this or did that. I had pizza for lunch. I'm waiting."

Then I'd get my hope right back up. That happened maybe fifty times in the course of one year.

You have to manage your recovery, which is long, slow, boring, confining and isolating; gradually re-enter; and then, often as not, go right back through the whole thing two weeks later. Sometimes a single joint would bleed and sort of heal and then bleed again, and then sort of heal and then bleed again. Every one of those bleedings during its reabsorbtion period was eating away at the joint so that eventually it wouldn't work and my muscles would atrophy. So after each bleeding, my joint was becoming more corroded and my muscles were getting weaker.

It was a very, very hard spiral to stop.

I think the important thing is that I came through all of this. I grew up.

I know that the way health insurance works in the United States is it gives the best coverage at the lowest cost to the people who need it least, and that, in fact, it is designed to exclude people who actually need medical care. I think that's disgraceful. That conviction comes out of my observations of this terrible, added burden that other people endure. They're already coping with an enormous amount, and then on top of that they're threatened with denial of care or with bankruptcy as a cost of trying to live through something over which they have no control. And that's in a country that normally commends itself for its compassion and good judgment. It's absolutely shocking. I like to make that point whenever I have the opportunity in the hope that someday the United States will set a different course.

One-on-one, I have benefited from a great many very serious, very compassionate, doctors and nurses. When I was a very young boy, a pediatrician named Mario Bisordi, who had sons with hemophilia, took care of me. Later I had Dr. Lee Engel in Westchester County, who would get up in the middle of the night, put on his clothes and a tie, get into his big, eight-cylinder car and drive over to give me a shot at three o'clock in the morning, Then he'd get back into his car, drive home and go to his practice the next day. That happened many, many, many times. Lee was always a wonderful, generous man. His partner, Dr. Herb Newman, was the same. That's the overarching thing.

For a long period in my adult life, I didn't have to go back to the hospital and when I started going back I was nervous about it because of the bad experiences. My wife reassured me. She said, "You know, Bob, things have changed and people are more responsive now."

I've definitely found that to be true. Part of it is also that I'm much smarter and more engaged and, as an adult, a more commanding patient.

What I'm proud of is my parents' decision to go ahead and write a book about our experiences as a family. I learned in the aftermath that for a period of ten to fifteen years, that book was very widely used in nursing schools. Even now, I occasionally get letters from people who talk about what an impact the book had.

It is possible to learn.

Reading my parents' book was a great revelation to me. Rereading it when I was myself a parent was probably the most revelatory moment, because I suddenly thought, "Oh, my God! How would I feel if this was happening to my son, Sam, or my son, John, or my daughter, Kate?" I realized that I have no idea whether I would react with the kind of strength and tenacity that my parents displayed. Reading it as a man in my thirties, when I had small children, taught me more about my parents than I thought I could learn. Because I'd grown up with them, I thought I knew all about them. But no, I learned a lot of new things.

My mother is a great lioness of support and my father, in a slightly quieter way, also, absolutely. That's a story in itself, how with such engaged parents, we were able to make separate lives. I think we negotiated that really, really well, partly because my parents, especially my mother, had a lot of other things she wanted to do, too. My mother became an international expert and historian on Russia. She wasn't sitting there saying, "You're my whole life." She was saying, "You are absolutely central to me, you and your sisters, and I can't wait for the moment when you have your independence, which we're all working for, and I can do more of the things that I'm interested in."

I was always relieved in a way that my mother and father, but especially, I think, my mother, had this whole set of aspirations and desires and interests. "Thank God. That means it's not all on me."

When I was four or five, we went up to Smith College. The day before we left, I was pushed against a doorknob by a classmate in nursery school. I got a bruise on my back and the bruise got worse as we drove north. And it got worse and worse and worse. In the middle of the night, it was huge. I couldn't move, so they took me to the hospital. Of course, this hospital in Northampton didn't have any fresh frozen plasma and they couldn't get it quickly, so my father lay down and gave whole blood.

One of the very vivid memories of my childhood is my big, strong daddy lying down, then the nurses drawing blood out of him and giving it to me.

When I was twelve, two things happened that had an extraordinary impact. One was that in 1968 I was taught to self-infuse. I still remember the nurse who taught me, a woman named Elaine Sergis, the nurse practitioner at New York Hospital. She also taught my father how to infuse, so sometimes my father would do it; sometimes I would do it under his supervision. Gradually, I gained the ability.

Secondly, the factor VIII concentrates began to appear. These made an enormous difference because not only were they much more powerful, but the key piece there for me was that the concentrates could be kept cool rather than frozen. That opened up an absolutely enormous vista for me to do things on my own, because I could take my bottles of factor with me.

Eventually they learned that the factor could be kept at room temperature and that meant that instead of being tethered to a hospital or to a large heavy-duty freezer, I could quite literally pack a backpack and go. I was able to give myself shots on camping trips or in the bathroom of an airborne 747.

Just at the moment of adolescence, when your life is expanding anyway, my ability to manage hemophilia improved in a way that allowed me this freedom. I was also regaining my ability to walk steadily.

There was an explosion from childhood to adulthood, a period that really went all the way through 1982 or 1983. I went to college. I went to divinity school. I was ordained in the Episcopal Church in 1982 and married in November of that year to my first wife, who is a religious historian and an incredibly talented woman. So the period from becoming a teenager — let's say in '72, '73 — to getting married in '82, was a period of enormous freedom for me.

Then, in 1984, I found out that I had HIV.

In 1984, when they had the antibody test, I discovered that I was HIV positive. This was before they had counseling or anything like that. I went for my annual check-up at New York Hospital, where they ran a battery of tests on me, checked all my joints and basically said, "How are you doing?" And I'd say, "I'm okay." Then they'd say, "Well, you know, you're doing pretty well compared to a lot of folks," and give me some advice like this: "Well, just keep it up, don't do too much, but keep going." People were very nice and I was glad to be checked from head to toe.

I know from subsequent events that the possibility that I might have contracted HIV was much more on the mind of my first wife than on mine and that she worried about this with gradually increasing intensity.

Our marriage ended in the early '90s, and I think that her concern was a major reason. I fault myself in some ways for not being more aware. I was operating on the basis of, "Well, we don't have any bad news and, you know, so far, so good," where she was operating from, "Oh, my goodness! This is a cloud on the horizon that's getting closer and closer."

Dr. Margaret Hilgartner, an incredible leader in the field out of New York Hospital, had been my caregiver since I was six or seven years old, and here I was twenty-eight when I found out about the HIV. I remember going into Margaret's office. She was always very good about asking me to step in and talk to her.

I remember Margaret saying, "Well, you know, we've run all these tests. Your liver functions are a little elevated," which I heard every time. We now understand that as a sign that my liver was deteriorating from hepatitis.

And then, as sort of an afterthought, she said, "Oh, do you want to know about the HIV score?" And I said, "Sure."

I remember her getting two books out. One was the list with my name and my subject number. The other showed my subject number and the result.

And she said, "Oh, well, you're positive."

I did not have any strong reaction. I didn't know what it meant. I basically went, "Oh?" And she sort of went, "Oh," and we agreed to "keep an eye on this." And I walked out. I really have to say I didn't give it that much thought. I said to myself, "All right, well, one more thing to keep an eye on."

I remember once being in a supermarket and looking down the aisle and seeing the checkout counter where they had the magazines. From forty feet away, I could see the cover of *Life* magazine, with a heading in huge red letters — I mean, you know, six-inch letters — "AIDS". The subtitle was, "Now, No One Is Safe." And I suddenly thought, "Oh-oh. Maybe I'm in real trouble."

I think there is a theme that runs through my life. One challenge, I think, for any person with a chronic illness, and particularly with hemophilia and with HIV, is to sense how much these phenomena that overtake you are going to affect your relationship with other people.

In the case of hemophilia, I had to work with all of the challenges and prejudices and anxieties that other people felt towards people with chronic illness, and particularly with braces. And then when HIV came along, there was that subtitle, "Now, no one is safe." I began to wonder whether I would have to start concealing my HIV status from people.

I think I'd always taken the point of view that hemophilia was ultimately not a frightening illness, that most of the things people were frightened about were not true. Once people's familiarity rose, their anxiety dropped, but HIV had these extremely emotional and panic-inducing qualities. It touched many of the most sensitive areas in people's mental and emotional makeup.

During this period, Dana and I were trying to decide what to do about having children. I was admitted to the Harvard Business School in the doctoral program with a full scholarship. I was always interested in economic and justice issues. We started talking about whether to have children then and we went through a very, very long process. I thought we were painstakingly thorough in trying to review all the emotional issues, the medical issues, the spiritual issues. Everything we could think of, we put on the table. I was apparently completely healthy. We didn't know much about the transition — it seemed like it was a small risk, so maybe we should try.

Dana got pregnant extremely quickly. Dana was fine, no trace of HIV, Sam was fine, and I said, "Thank you, God." And I thought, "Well, maybe that's all we'll do." I thought "Phew, that's enough. I'm fine. I'm happy and thank you." The decision to have John was something of an impulse. Dana said, "I want to have a child, like, right now," and she did. The sad part of this story is that despite the courage she showed, her sense that my life was going to definitely be foreshortened continued to gnaw at her. That part was very, very hard for her. It wore away and led to the end of our marriage.

If I had to pick out difficult times from among all the things that I've been through, that was probably the hardest thing in my whole life.

On the positive side, we had these two beautiful boys.

One thing I learned is that there's always a bias against safety, because people want to move a product out and they don't want to hear bad news. I think there's no question that, in this instance, and in other instances that followed, commerce overwhelmed science and did end up exposing a great many people, including me. Not to put too fine a point on it, if in response to the hepatitis concerns that were already well-established in the mid-1970s, the pharmaceutical companies had decided to pursue a system of viral inactivation or heat treatment, there would have been no HIV catastrophe for the hemophilia community. That speaks for itself.

Your success in life, your access to basic forms of care, whether it's a good doctor or a good home, or even a good job, should not be determined by your connections. Unless we have a system that is powerfully committed to inclusion and to equity, you are going to end up with a system that distributes benefits according to connections and not according to need or according to fairness. It is a constant struggle in America as to which image of life is going to dominate. Is it the one where there's a basic sense of justice, inclusion and fairness, where people who are not to blame for the things that have happened to them are given access to the resources to survive and to succeed? Or is it just going to be a lottery, where some people have crushing things happen to them and are simply wiped out, while other people are born to privilege and never have to think about another thing.

The America that I know and love and that I think people admire is the first one, not the second.

I think the forces of hatred, homophobia, the people who predicted that HIV was a plague brought on by an alien group who needed to be isolated, all failed in the broad sense. Sadly, for individual people there were still pockets of bigotry and brutality that continued. We can't say that America escaped completely, but the weight of public judgment — the actors and actresses, other public leaders who stepped forward and were willing to identify with people with HIV — really helped. That was a moment when America could have become something truly horrible and chose not to; it chose to be compassionate.

I was awestruck by the love, patience, compassion and commitment demonstrated by many members of the gay community towards people in other groups with HIV. I watched gay men give of themselves to other people through the most painful of circumstances and with a strength that any human being would be proud and touched to see.

In political terms, I think it is totally unacceptable to have a system in which not only do we have widespread poverty and disease, but also in which we blame poverty on the poor and we blame suffering and disability on the diseased, as though we still have this early Biblical mentality that holds that if you are having so much trouble, it must be because of something you did wrong. Now, of course, people make mistakes and can intensify their own problems. I absolutely believe that one needs to mobilize one's own sense of responsibility and agency and move out of victimhood and into strength, but one of the ways you do that is that others provide you with resources and affirm that you can do it.

I was exposed from a very early age to something about as close to unconditional love as you can get in this life from other people. My parents loved me unquestioningly. Their support for me was so overwhelming that during the moments when I was the most exposed or in pain or in danger, I never doubted them. In the many things that I had to fear, the one thing I didn't have to fear was the withdrawal of their love. I think that set up a core set of convictions about the power of love and about my own self-worth, which was an essential ingredient in everything I was able to do and be afterwards.

When I wasn't able to walk, the highest aspiration of my whole life was that I would be able to walk again. Now that I can walk, I don't want to be one of these people who says, "Well, thank you, and now that I've got the highest aspiration of my whole life, I have a new list of highest aspirations of my whole life." Well, of course you do. That's what human beings do. But even as I move on, I need to remember that I achieved the highest aspiration of my life.

I sometimes think, "What kind of person would I have been if I hadn't had hemophilia?" Some things probably would have been very much the same: my energy and enthusiasm and curiosity and so forth. But I think the arrogance would have been much greater.

That's not to say I'm without arrogance now. I might have wanted to become a fighter pilot or an astronaut or a hotshot, and, you know, it would have been fun to go zooming around and be a tough guy. What I realized was that I so easily could have been a straight, white, privileged male in the dominant country of its era in some position of great authority and wealth, and that I could have achieved all of those things. And my predominant response could have been, "I did it. Why couldn't everybody else?"

One of the mysteries discussed a lot in the Bible is how is it that good fortune produces hardness of heart? It doesn't always, but you would think that the more good things that happen to people, the more humble and generous they would be. In fact, very often, the more that good things happen to people, the more judgmental they become of people to whom bad things have happened, and the more tightly they control what they have.

That response is mysterious to me.

I think in the first instance, when you're talking to a family that's confronting hemophilia, the first thing is to help them grieve.

We go through life building up elaborate senses of what the future is going to be like, how we will get there and how we deserve that. I use the term "pictures in the head." Losing the pictures in the head — and the sense of the narrative of your life — is very painful. In fact, one Catholic writer defines that loss as the essence of suffering. Pain is one thing, but suffering is the loss of a narrative that gives your life meaning.

The first thing is to help people step through the sorrow about the fact that whatever it was that they imagined, may not happen. That's part of growing up. The second piece is that you're not going to lose everything. Many of the things that you think right now are going to be gone for good are, in fact, probably still going to happen. Then you start being able to say things like, "And the care is so much better," and, you know, "A child can achieve autonomy." So the things that one longs for in a child, which is to free the child from suffering and to enable that child to grow into a full, happy and free individual, are all still possible for both the child and for you as a parent. Many, many things that can happen, will happen.

Another thing I would say is focus on this cushion of unconditional love. That is the greatest tool you can give to a child, especially one who's coping with a chronic illness. That doesn't mean you have to be perfect or that you have to always be loving. You can be strong and you can provide guidance on proper behavior and discipline when necessary. But the core idea is that we don't love you any less because of what you're going through.

I guess the final thing is to mobilize the resources that are out there, and to recognize that one is not lost in some isolation, but that there's a community of people who have experience and resources who are willing to help you out. The only thing that will deny you access to that is your own decision to remain isolated. If you remain frightened and withdrawn, then you cut off the ability of so many others to provide you with what you need. Isolation is a danger with all kinds of suffering.

It was a great trial when I was divorced. Essentially what happened is that the person I trusted to love me unconditionally and forever — the picture in my head — suddenly announced that she didn't. I think there was a real question in my mind for a while as to whether I could make sense of it all and find love again. I did and I have an incredible wife, Anne, who had been a friend of mine before and had not married.

No matter how hard we work at it, I don't think we can guarantee that our human relationships are all going to work out. My experience was a kind of death followed by a kind of resurrection into a new life of love and comfort and mutual support.

I love being a father. I don't pretend to understand how my children have internalized or made sense of all the medical problems I face. In one sense, I'm candid about them and those issues are part of our daily life. They've seen me have shots. They know when I have a bandage on my arm. They know this.

My daughter Kate, who's six, divided her engagement with me into things that she can do with me now, and things that she will be able to do with me after my liver transplant. My son John is incredibly into sports and, of course,

I have virtually no experience playing sports. We tease about this. The little fiction we have going is that, in fact, I was a great sports hero, that I won the Heisman Trophy, that I was drafted for the NBA and I had to pick between that and my stellar baseball career. We'll be watching some old Celtics player and John will say, "Oh, you must remember him from your days, Dad." And I say, "Yes, I taught him everything he knows."

We joke about that and it's quite funny as a running joke, both of us imagining me as a running back or as a shortstop. It's fun for me to think about it; it's fun for him to think about it. It means that we can embrace it.

And there's another thing that I just want to mention, which is that right now, even as we're talking, I'm going through a most amazing experience — one of the most amazing experiences of my life, because for me to have a new life, restored energy and, possibly, literally curing my hemophilia, I need to go through a liver transplant from a living donor.

The pictures in my head are a little fuzzy right now as to what the future represents, but I may be able to go on to new things, things that are unimaginable right now. I have survived HIV for reasons that are absolutely unclear. I have had HIV for twenty-six years, for more than half my life, and I'm still here drawing breath and enjoying my life. And now you add to that the fact that somebody may give up a portion of his own liver in order to give me an extended life and to free me permanently from hemophilia. That's just an amazing story. And what kind of life should flow from that? It seems to me somehow a life of great rejoicing and great generosity.

If I had the time and energy to move forward, what I would want to be able to do is to give people hope, because we live in a world where people try to steal or crush each other's hope all the time. Even through all these difficult things, I have had this opportunity to go into worlds that are better, and I think we can do that as a community, too.

Even if this all ends not really that well — let's say I don't get a transplant, or I get it and it doesn't work — I'm really not at all afraid of the future, because I feel my life has been so unbelievably rich, even with all the challenges, right up to now. None of that can be taken away. It's all part of who I am and what I've been able to do and who I've been able to love and care about, and that's all been completed. It exists already in its fullness. So we're talking about adding to that.

A part of me believes that you're a stronger person and more honest with yourself if you've really embraced the hard times, if you've cried for yourself.

Mark Borreliz

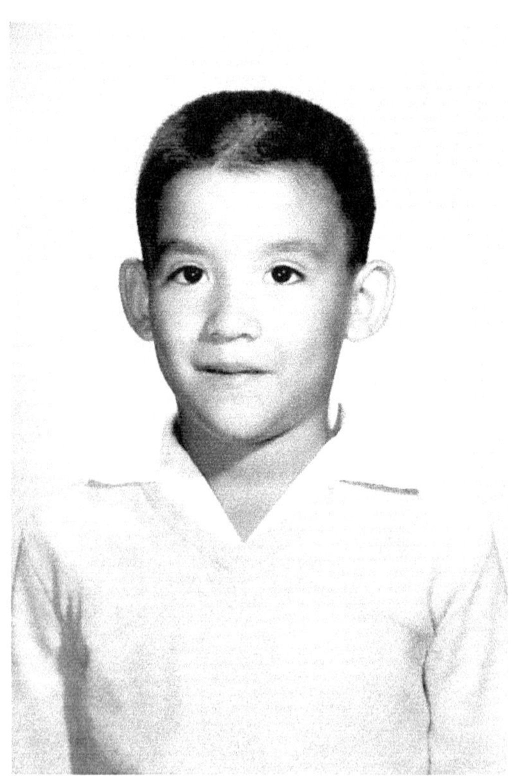

Mark's 2nd grade school photo, 1959.

MARK BORRELIZ

Mark Borreliz was born in 1952 on a U.S. Army base in Albuquerque, New Mexico. He is married and has two children. Mark attended Harvard College and Law School and practiced law in Boston for more than twenty years. He has severe factor VIII deficiency and is a long-term HIV survivor. At one time infected with hepatitius C, he eliminated the virus in 2003. Mark retired from full-time legal practice in 2001 due to health issues and now devotes his time to writing, painting and volunteer work for various organizations, including the New England Hemophilia Association.

Violating household rules in my house was easy, and that put a curious twist on growing up as a hemophiliac. With my mother, almost anything you did that deviated from the norm was cause for scrutiny, if not discipline. One of the things I did periodically was injure myself, and I always dreaded the injury coming to light because with my mother, there was always a mix of anger and, of course, maternal attentiveness. There was always that blend, and I grew up hiding a lot of my injuries.

I don't know quite what my parents made of my hemophilia. I think there was some feeling that my mother had given me this. My father has never been clear on it, other than feeling badly. He's never indicated how he felt, but I'm sure he was mystified and didn't know quite what to do.

My mother went into a very protective mode. I grew up being told, "You shouldn't have been with that friend. You should have known better than to do this or that." I feel as though that attitude did me some harm over the years, instilling in me a sense of fragility. On the positive side, my mother's overreaction put into place policies that got me through to adulthood.

In the '50s and continuing into the early '60s, the treatment for a bleed—if it was a serious bleed and required hospitalization—was to be placed almost instantly on bed rest. To stop the bleeding, they gave whole blood or fresh frozen plasma.

From an early age, I was used to the idea of having one arm or the other strapped to a board, being immobilized, then having an IV set up. I stayed that way for several days. Eventually, the whole contraption was shifted to the other arm.

I still remember finally having my arm unstrapped and the terrible painfulness of bending that arm for the first time. And, of course, there weren't those wonderful, plastic-tipped catheters then, so you really had to keep the arm straight. If you moved it too much, you felt the needle point.

I'll tell you a story that saddens me.

When I was five, I developed terrible cavities in several of my molars and they decided that the molars should be extracted. As it turned out, I was hospitalized for six weeks, and during that time I only saw my mother once. I remember feeling like an orphan.

The extractions were performed under some form of general anesthesia and, after the teeth were out, I bled a lot. I was on a liquid diet for a long time and I was even fed through a tube for a while.

When the naso-gastric tube was put in, I had no idea what it was. Army hospitals didn't make a big point of explaining things to kids. A couple of nurses and orderlies appeared at the bed, my limbs were pinned down and somebody would proceed to insert these tubes. My gag reflex was working mightily and I was fighting it. Eventually the tube was in and I lived with that for a while.

There were moments during that hospital admission when I felt very alone. I would wake up in the middle of the night with my mouth literally filled with sacks of blood, clots the size of ping pong balls, or so they felt. They were big enough that I couldn't even move my tongue to talk, so when I wanted to get someone's attention, I made bleating noises. A nurse would appear and cut the clots off and the process would begin again.

In the end, it was just another bunch of experiences. I didn't feel oppressed or incarcerated, I simply felt apart from my family and off on something of an adventure that had its mean times and its exhilarating times.

Often I was surprised to find that there were compassionate people, people who were good with kids. For those people, I was immensely grateful.

I never saw hemophilia as something that was preventing me from achieving the important things in life. Isn't that amazing, even though in school it meant there was no PE for me whatsoever? I might accompany the class and watch them at PE. I might keep score for their games. I might carry the equipment. None of that made me feel like a second-class citizen. It actually made me feel as though I was part of it.

Here's the way in which I feel extraordinarily lucky. For whatever reason, I was easygoing and I had a sense of humor. I think that helped a lot. I always fit in, although all my friends knew that I had a bleeding disease and that I couldn't do a lot of things. Most of all, I think I always had a sense of humor, and it's amazing to me how you can build relationships on that.

In spite of everything, my mother expected that I would do well in school and that I would never be a disciplinary problem. That had to be squared with my hemophilia. I'm sure she agonized much more than I'll ever know. As a parent now, I have a much greater understanding of her feelings, and I'm sure she felt terrific guilt for having been a carrier of this illness.

As a child, pain was an episodic event, and sometimes they were quite extraordinary episodes. Taking care of the pain meant keeping an ice pack on my foot twenty-four hours a day, removing the pack only when the foot was totally numb and blue.

I think maybe I have a different view of pain because of what happened to me. I'm not scared of pain, and a big component of pain, of course, is fear — fear of what else is coming; fear of what the pain signifies. It helps if I understand the mechanism and know that the pain is not going to go out of control. Pain is something I have a pretty good tolerance for, I think.

A part of me believes that you're a stronger person and more honest with yourself if you've really embraced the hard times, if you've cried for yourself.

I remember hours of lying in a hospital bed as a kid studying patterns in the ceiling tiles. There must have been a lot of thinking done, because I'm still very comfortable with quiet, contemplative time. It's always a bit of a treasure to me. I think I developed a real patience then.

Many times I have found myself trying to reassure my parents that the reality they projected onto the situation wasn't quite right. Kids have an astonishing ability to cope with what's going on around them, to be all right with things as they are, to find in whatever confines are left to them, some diversions that are completely, thoroughly engaging.

It's a great thing, thank goodness.

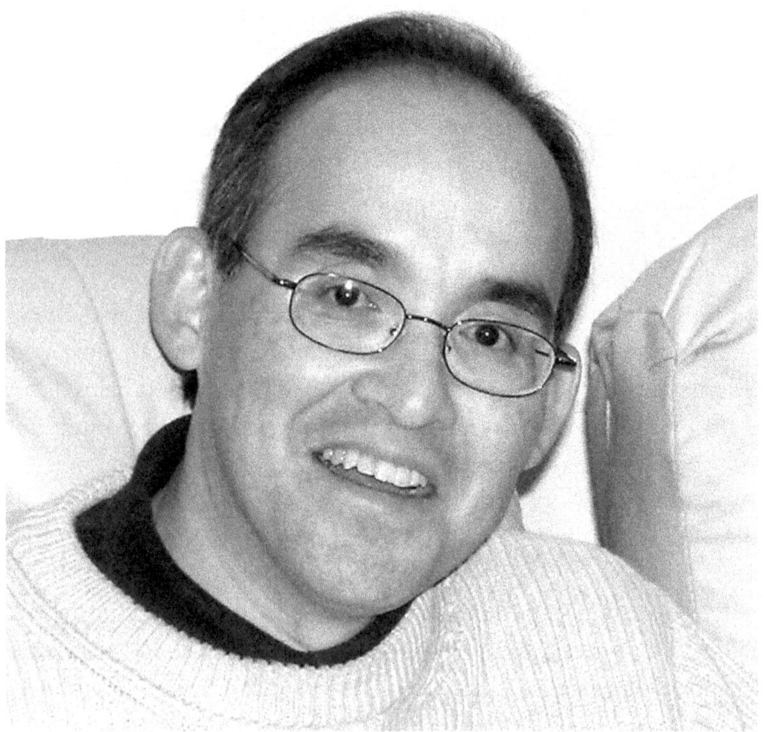

Mark Borreliz

When I first received cryoprecipitate, it was fantastic. It seemed like a relatively small volume of plasma, and I wasn't expecting it to be very effective. I went to sleep that night thinking, "Tomorrow morning I'm still going to be on bed rest for a few days," and I was amazed. It was a miracle to wake up with no pain in my ankle and next to no pain in my elbow.

"Wow," I thought, "it must be because I was hoping so desperately to be better this morning."

For a little while, there was the notion that all the hemophiliacs who were testing positive for the viral antibody had, in fact, developed antibodies that had the effect of actually immunizing one against HIV. There was even the thought that in the hemophilia population, being "positive" meant something different than it did in the gay population or for drug users.

That idea faded quickly.

My wife and I were married in 1987. We both knew I had HIV, but we wanted to have children. We knew there was an HIV transmission risk, but we didn't have much by way of statistical information available to us. The data just weren't there yet. We contacted the Hemophilia Treatment Center in Worcester, and they had a handful of couples who had successfully had children without transmitting HIV to the wife or children. Based on that near-anecdotal information, we had our first child in 1989.

We're both pretty cautious people. It's amazing to me that we went ahead.

In the early '90s, I believed that I was not going to see my children grow up. Those were very grim years, with these two little kids I was nuts about, as any new parent is. I remember lying awake at night and grieving a little bit for what I would not see.

It's ironic, of course, that hemophiliacs have normal children. I'm now raising a twelve-year-old son who happens to have chosen gymnastics as his passion. He already has, at this stage, upper body strength that exceeds mine.

"Well, Daddy is the guy who runs three steps before he has to infuse." Or, "Well, he's not going to do too many chin-ups. On one of them he's going to leave his left arm hanging from the bar because of that artificial elbow." We joke about it all the time, but the reality is there's a great irony in raising a physically fit, if not extra-athletic, son. That's a bit of a challenge and fun. There are ways to do it right, and I don't think it needs to be hard. The contrast is just a curious feature that comes of being a parent with hemophilia.

By the time I was a young lawyer, I was in a terrible state as far as some of my joints were concerned. I endured daily pain for years in my knee. There was bone on bone, no cartilage any more to cushion the joint, and every step hurt like the dickens. I was using crutches, canes, sometimes walkers, and trying to conduct a legal practice.

To get to a meeting a block and a half away, I would set out about half an hour ahead. I cut a very pathetic figure, moving very slowly down the block.

I was sitting on top of a fantastic, satisfying legal practice, watching my CD4 levels drop and my viral load sky-rocket. Finally, I was advised by a very caring and inimitable doctor that I had to choose now. I had to choose between continuing to be a big-city, high-powered lawyer for a short while or having a life that went on for a longer time. I still marvel that after I was told this, I walked out of that appointment, went back to my office and proceeded to shut my practice down.

As far as the clinicians who were sued, I think that's a great misfortune because the caregivers I met in the hemophilia community were not motivated by the need to push tainted blood products. That would be inimical to their nature and motivations. I've never met a clinician in the hemophilia community who didn't have the loftiest intentions and the most caring and kindest orientation you could ask for.

In the end, I received one of those hundred thousand dollar settlements. How little that is in terms of a life valuation. Well, it hasn't cost me my life, but it has cost me my career, and it's put me in the realm of living very carefully and putting up with the daily vexations of the HIV meds.

I'm inclined to feel in my gut that the drug companies did get away with something, and I took some pretty short dollars in exchange for it, but I don't dwell on that.

One's life as a physician, working with hemophilia, is a series of stories. Every patient has a story about his hemophilia, what it's meant to him and his family. You get close to the people who are living that life, and you can't help but get wrapped up in it.

If you don't get wrapped up in it, you're a stone.

Dr. Gilbert White

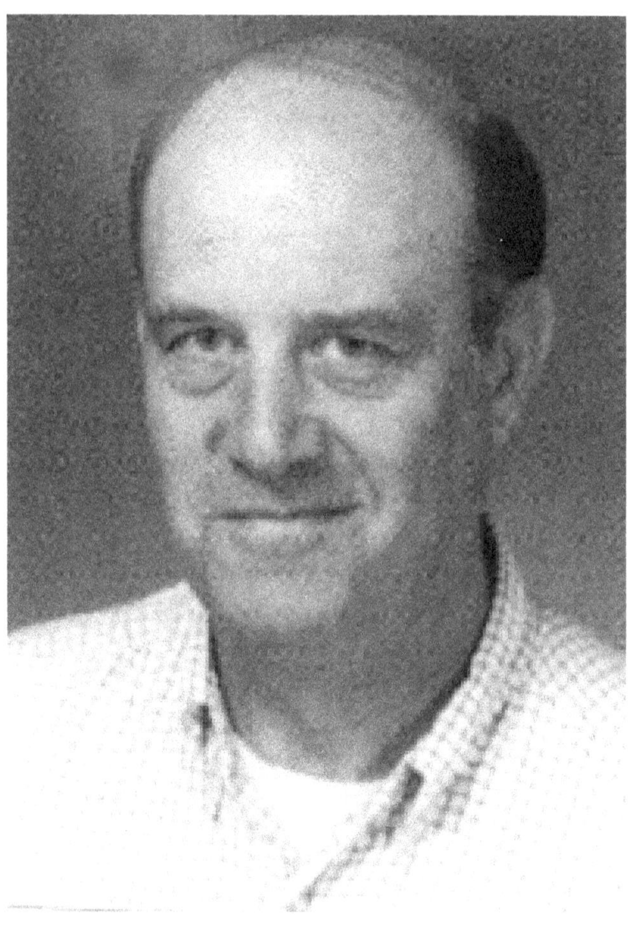

Dr. Gilbert White

DR. GILBERT C. WHITE

Dr. Gilbert C. White is currently the Executive Vice President for Research at the BloodCenter of Wisconsin and the Director of BloodCenter's Blood Research Institute in Milwaukee, Wisconsin. He was previously the Director of the Harold R. Roberts Comprehensive Hemophilia Treatment Center and the Director of the Center for Thrombosis and Hemostasis at the University of North Carolina at Chapel Hill from 1988 to 2004. Dr. White is married and has three children and two grandchildren.

Looking back over thirty years of treating patients with hemophilia, you realize what a special population of patients they are, and you realize what they've gone through. Taking care of the same people for thirty years is an amazing experience. In the latter part of my career, I was seeing their grandsons, or maybe even their great-grandsons, and that's an experience! It isn't something that you see with many diseases. This was real family-based medicine.

Working with the hemophilia population was also comprehensive medicine. If you took care of a patient with hemophilia, you had to know psychiatry, you had to know liver disease, you had to know infectious diseases. These patients also got heart disease and cancer, so it was total medicine in the sense that you had to be a good general practitioner in taking care of all the different aspects. You had to know what hepatitis was and how to treat it, what AIDS was and how to treat it, what depression was and how to treat it, and so on.

There are a lot of memories. I remember a lot of the early patients and the bad joint disease they had. I remember the first transfusion of recombinant factor VIII, given in Chapel Hill, and I was lucky enough to be there. I still remember the patient quite well, a person with whom I still talk often.

We wanted the first patient to be a good spokesperson for hemophilia, a positive- thinking person, somebody who knew what plasma transfusions were like, what cryoprecipitate was like, what the first concentrates were like, what transfusion-transmitted diseases were like. This was an older individual who had been through a lot, who had experienced earlier treatment, a person who'd known death in his family due to hemophilia, a person who had joint disease because he hadn't been able to give himself treatment, someone who antedated home therapy.

The occasion actually produced a humorous story. I remember, we were giving the first infusion of recombinant factor VIII in the clinical research unit and there were TV cameras. It was a very serious occasion, and we didn't know what was going to happen with the infusion of this material.

I'd spent a lot of time telling this individual what the material was, how it had been made in Chinese hamster ovary cells and that it had been genetically engineered. I told him I wasn't sure it was folded right, and that he might develop an inhibitor as a result.

There were bright lights and it was kind of hot; I was nervous, and I think the nurse was nervous. I was infusing the material, but the patient's eyes were closed and his head was sort of leaning back. Let's say his name was Fred, and I whispered "Fred, are you okay?" He didn't say anything, so I said it a little louder.

"Fred, are you okay?"

And all of a sudden he started making hamster noises!

"I'm turning into a hamster!" he said.

So we were very nervous, but obviously he was very relaxed.

Fred was potentially interested in gene therapy. The real point of the story is that after the product was approved, Genetics Institute invited Fred to come up to the research headquarters. There was a spiral staircase with a landing halfway up, and Gabe Schmergel, the head of the company, went up to the first landing to make some comments. The whole company was gathered down below.

"This is a momentous occasion," he said. "We have approval for this product, and recombinant factor VIII will now be available for use by hemophiliacs."

He asked Fred if he would like to make some comments.

Fred has terrible joint disease, but he walked up those steps to the landing. When he got up there, he told a story about how his brother had died at an early age. He talked about some of the things that had happened to him, and how much it meant that recombinant factor VIII, a safe form of factor VIII, would now be available for hemophiliacs. Fred had the whole place in tears! It was really an amazing and wonderful story.

I don't know how Fred got up to the landing. From what people told me, you could have heard a pin drop in that place while he was walking up the stairs. Fred got up there and said some profound things. You can't help but feel some level of gratification. I'm not gratified that people died, but I'm thankful that I was a part of the hemophilia experience, that I was able to see some of the things that people did, and the way they responded — patients and health care workers, families and brothers and sisters.

One's life as a physician, working with hemophilia, is a series of stories. Every patient has a story about his hemophilia, what it's meant to him and his family. You get close to the people who are living that life, and you can't help but get wrapped up in it.

If you don't get wrapped up in it, you're a stone.

There's a lot of addiction to pain medications in hemophilia. You want to relieve their pain, but you don't want them to become addicted, and you don't know how to do it. I mean, there are no magic bullets. You want to make their pain go away, but you don't want to turn them into helpless addicts, either. So, you know, you get terribly involved emotionally in that kind of a decision.

Sometimes you're so involved that you probably don't make the right decision; for example, you might give the patient more pain medication than he ought to have because of his story. Hemophilia is a very human disease; it's not the same as a patient you see for two years then it's over. This is someone you've seen for thirty years! You know all their warts. You know all their good points. You see them as kids, with all their hopes. You know the things they've triumphed over. You know the things that have beaten them down. You are uplifted when they do something they didn't think they could do, and you are crushed when they can't do something they wanted to do.

From a doctor's point of view, hemophilia is a pretty remarkable disease. I see these patients from birth to death, and they become like my own family.

People throw the word "heroes" around a lot. I don't think those men with hemophilia and then hepatitis and HIV thought of themselves as heroes. They thought of themselves as people who had something put upon them that they didn't put upon themselves, but they are heroes, in a way. Some got angry and lashed out, and some just tried to go about living their lives. Everybody responded differently to HIV and hepatitis C, but they all lived with it.

They all did whatever it was they were going to do.

Many didn't make it. I sat in a room with a twenty-one-year-old fellow who died of a combination of HIV and liver disease. He was bleeding all over the room, and throwing up blood, and it was an unforgettable experience from many perspectives. It was also unforgettable because this was somebody I had known and cared a great deal about for fifteen years, and to see him having to go through that was hard. I wrote a letter to his parents a week ago; they are the greatest people in the world.

I have a piece that that young man wrote and gave to me a couple of weeks before he died. He'd just graduated from college and had a girlfriend, and they were talking about getting married. He gave this to me, but I think it was written to his fiancée.

"As we all know," he wrote, "anything that has an origin also has an ending. It seems so hard sometimes to understand why, yet I do feel that the acceptance stage must be a realization of death, and not a surrendering to it, the fight for life and the quality thereof. It's a shame that you have to be confronted with death to appreciate life: the smile on a child's face, a fresh bouquet of flowers, getting caught in the rain, sand washing under your feet as the tide begins its monotonous journey back to base.

"You would think we were all comfortable enough with death and dying that going to the alabaster palace would be inviting. So why must we mourn the passage when it should be a celebration more important than graduation, marriage, and retirement combined? When I do go, I hope it does not entail my suffering and wasting away.

"I love you and I guess if I do go early, I'll get the place ready for you when you arrive. Who knows? Maybe I'll get to be an influence in your life down the road.

"My life didn't turn out the way I had originally planned, but I had a great family and friends to help. No one truly gets what they want, but if you always keep an open mind and a positive attitude, it makes the ride easier. I hope I move up a notch or two in the food chain. This is the end, my friend, my only friend. Begin again."

Twenty-one. Twenty-one years old, a young guy, and very talented.

I don't think I ever showed those patients my true emotions — hardly ever — but the emotions were there, and my patients were the reason for them. When I was in the room with this kid? I mean, there was no way I couldn't have shown it. By being there, I was showing my emotions, but, I mean, you don't show it the way a parent does, because you're not a parent. You don't show it in the same way you might for your brother, because the patient is not your brother. As the doctor, you're supposed to be more of a steadying influence.

I've said that the patients were heroes, but to me, the real heroes of that time were the nurses. The two nurses we had at the UNC Center are just really outstanding people. They weren't beaten down by it; they didn't get depressed. They kept moving forward; they remained positive. I don't know how they did it. They had to deal with the patients much more directly than physicians did, and I know that's true at every center.

The nurses were the people who provided the sympathy the patients needed, and that took an awful lot out of the nurses. You only have so much sympathy to dole out in your lifetime, and I know that my two nurses used up an awful lot of that sympathy. They were great.

I think the nurses are pretty amazing people. They're all dedicated. I know my two nurses, Aime and Brenda, well and I think they're the best, but I've been impressed with the quality of nursing in hemophilia throughout the world. A lot of nurses from other countries have come to Chapel Hill to learn, and their dedication and commitment is impressive. I've known nurses at other centers, and they're just as dedicated. I don't know whether the disease attracts that kind of dedication, or whether it's just something that human beings do when they're confronted with the sort of situations that hemophilia presents. I think it's the latter, because I don't see otherwise how you could get such a committed group attracted to the care of one disease.

I guess people just adapt to doing the right thing sometimes. There are some bad people in the world, and there are some good people in the world, and I think most of the nurses that are in the hemophilia centers are just the good people in the world.

Aime Grimsley's been here about eighteen years, and Brenda Nielsen about fifteen years, so their time as nurses with us goes way back. I had my lab to retreat to; that was my escape. They didn't have that. They went back to their office, where the phone would ring again, and somebody would say, "What do I do?" It was more of a battlefield for them, and I was more like a general who would make an appearance, then go back to the safety of my tent in the rear.

I don't think all nurses made it through. I think a lot of nurses were worn down, and dropped out. I can think of several nurses that I'm sure are doing what they're currently doing because they just couldn't keep dealing with it. I also think they did their nursing largely without support — I mean, other than the support that I could give them, and that they could give each other, and the rewards that the patients gave them.

That is the ultimate nursing reward, the ultimate physician reward, the reward that your patients give you, and I think our patients were appropriately grateful for what the nurses did.

We knew what HIV was, but we still didn't necessarily know what you had to do to get rid of it. Until the identification of that virus as the causative agent, we didn't even have a *bona fide* way of testing for it. You had surrogate methods, like T-4 cells, but people who have hepatitis have decreased T-4 cells, too, so just measuring T-4 cells didn't really tell you whether they had HIV or not. So, you knew, and you didn't know.

This was before we knew that HIV was a virus, before we knew that it was HIV, and we didn't know how to kill it.

Companies introduced heat-treated factor as a way of eliminating hepatitis. Well, it didn't get rid of hepatitis; it got rid of HIV. People were grabbing at anything to try and get rid of this infectious material. All the studies at the CDC supported the fact that it was a blood-borne infectious agent, so you knew you had to do something to the blood to get rid of it. Some centers were going to cryoprecipitate. Some centers were using heat-treated. Some centers were saying, "Don't treat." I mean, here we are going back to the beginning of hemophilia care: don't treat. Suffer.

Nobody knew what to do, and I honestly believe that in most cases people were innocent of any negligence — there just wasn't a clue as to what to do. I talked a lot with my colleagues, and I know that MASAC did a lot of talking about what to do, and I think, in the end, heat treatment wound up being the thing that saved some people. The sad thing is that it just wasn't done quickly enough, but nobody knew.

Most of the people were infected with HIV before the first case of AIDS was even described! The first case of AIDS was described in '81, and most epidemiological retrospective studies suggest that people were infected as early as '78, '79 and '80. Concentrates were coming from those donors who hadn't yet manifested disease. In spite of that, there was a lot of guilt and a lot of anger.

What is so striking is that these men had suffered with virtually no treatment, or minimal treatment, for most of their lives. Then they take treatment, and they suffer for that. That is what makes hemophilia a special disease, the fact that they suffered before the concentrate and they suffered after the concentrate. At the same time, these patients are always positive, always looking for the next thing. That's what you have to do with a chronic disease, you stay positive and look for the next thing, and it'll come to you whether you look for it or not, because we're always making advances.

Gene therapy and stem cell therapy are the next hope. We were always very active in our Center in clinical trials because I wanted patients to have the option of being a part of developing the next treatment. They didn't have to volunteer for those trials, but we made the opportunity available if they wanted to partake in advancing the treatment of their own disease.

Nobody wants to see better treatments more than the people who have the diseases, and if they have an opportunity to participate in those studies, to be a part of the research, then that gives them hope. It gives them a reason to keep moving on, to keep looking down the road.

Money doesn't bring anybody back. When you get right down to it, I don't think money makes you feel any better, but it's something. A nation is defined by its compassion, and if a nation can't have the compassion to feel sorry for these patients, then there's something wrong with the nation. If they hadn't done Ricky Ray, there would have been something seriously wrong with this country. I mean, when you get past all the discussion and the talk and everything, that's what Ricky Ray is about. It's about asking the question, "Are we a compassionate nation?"

Or do we say, "You drew the short straw; no reason to give you anything."

I wrote an obituary for Kenneth Brinkhous, who died on December 11th, 2000, at age ninety-two. I think it's a little part of this oral history. In the first sentence I basically said that it's rare that a person sees a disease defined initially and then sees its cure. Kenneth Brinkhous came close to that experience with hemophilia.

There are some good things happening in the inhibitor and joint disease areas, too. I think people are really finally starting to focus again on those aspects of hemophilia. For twenty years, we focused on infectious complications, and now we're able to get back to the real issues, the issues we were trying to address from 1975 to 1981, the issues that we had to put aside for awhile.

There's something to be said for having some sense of history about things, a sense that gives you a human appreciation of where things have been, and where they are today. That's what an oral history is all about. I do think that history has a role.

My grandson, Eric, has hemophilia and when he has grown up and I'm gone, I hope that he gets a chance to ask some questions about Grandpa and how he dealt with things. I hope that something I did helps him understand that you can go ahead and do what you've got to do and live a life with God's help that is normal, just, good and in which you contribute.

You don't have to let this disease or anything else stop you.

Wendell Bourne

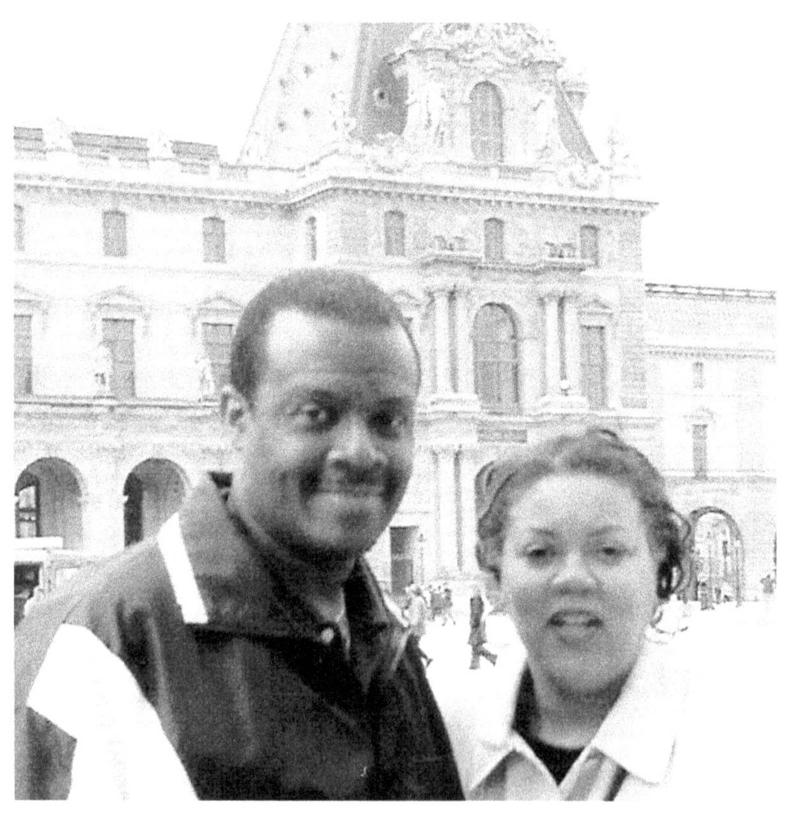

Wendell and his wife, Margo, in front of the Louvre during a vacation trip to Paris, April 2001.

WENDELL BOURNE

Mr. Wendell Bourne was born in 1948 in Cambridge, Massachusetts. He is married and has four children; his one grandson has hemophilia. Mr. Bourne is the Coordinator of History and Social Science education for kindergarten through 12th grade in the Cambridge school system. He is an African-American whose faith has been an enormous resource in handling life's challenges. He has severe factor VIII deficiency and hepatitis C.

Well, as the story goes, my mom said when I was really young they noticed a couple of little bruises, but it really wasn't something that concerned them at first. When I was about eighteen months old, I fell in my explorations around the house and hit my mouth. As she describes, it, I broke that little piece of skin just behind the upper lip and it started to bleed. Naturally, they applied ice and pressure, but it didn't stop. That's what sent us to the hospital, where the doctors also had some problems stopping the bleeding. They ran blood tests and that's when my hemophilia was diagnosed.

My mom, Abney Bourne, grew up in South Carolina, where her father and mother owned a 168-acre farm. Her father was a farmer and a preacher. There were five girls and two boys in the family. When my grandmother's family and my grandfather's family came together it constituted a huge number of people. They were growing up in the country during the early part of the twentieth century, so if there had been someone who lived only a portion of his life and died, it wouldn't have been particularly unusual. No one knew, nor was it determined, whether anyone had hemophilia.

You have to understand that health care in the south for African-Americans at that time was probably such that it was not likely that something like hemophilia would have been discovered and treated in the late 1800s or the early 1900s. If someone in the family, one of my ancestors, had hemophilia, we don't know.

My sense is that, for whatever reasons, my dad wasn't able to deal with my hemophilia. That might have been his way of distancing himself. I don't remember any conversations, encounters, connections with my dad and my disease. Most of my memories of in and out of the hospital in later years are just of my mom.

I remember coming into Emergency. We came in so often that a lot of the nurses and aides in there knew who we were; they knew me by name. In fact, my mom still knew these folks twenty, thirty years later. There was one woman working in there who, when I went in one day as an adult, recognized me and asked about my mom. We spent a lot of time in there. A lot of time.

The treatment at the time was frozen blood plasma. We spent hours in the emergency room while several of the thawed-out plastic bags of fresh frozen blood plasma were dripped in at a safe rate, so as not to cause reactions. I had a few "hive" reactions to some of this material when I was little. Once you got it in, you had to wait for the bleeding to recede. They had to keep a five-year-old quiet.

I had lots of casts, particularly casts that were cut in half with straps on them, so that you could take them off as the swelling went down. My leg was in casts for long periods. I was on crutches a lot for anything I whacked or banged.

When I was well enough to go back to school I would be on crutches and, you know, kids get out of your way and kind of give you all this, "Can we help?" and so forth. I became known as the sickly boy who was always on crutches.

I don't remember hemophilia dampening my spirit or my sense of adventure or my wanting to do different things.

Naturally, I couldn't play any sports in school, but I remember seeing the other kids playing. I don't remember a real active physical education experience in school because, if I was relatively healthy, they were afraid that something would happen to me. I never even tried out for anything. If I was on crutches, I didn't even have to go down to gym. I stayed in the room and read a book or did something else.

My mom always encouraged me to do different things short of organized sports. She got me involved in Cub Scouts and church activities. We were very involved in our church. Still are. In my adolescent years, she sent me off to Camp Caravan for kids with disabilities. You had kids in wheelchairs, kids on crutches, kids with braces, kids who looked normal but had other things going on. Oh, that was a ball. I was even elected mayor of Camp Caravan one year. I had my first little girlfriend. She gave me a kiss in the woods. These are things that you don't forget.

My mother always allowed me to experience things, but, at the same time, she was very protective. At home, sharp corners had little pads taped on them. Sharp objects or anything I could have bumped myself on were pushed aside. She was very conscious about that, even today. I'll be in my own house and I'll tap against something and Mom will say "You okay?" She still asks —"Hit yourself?"

"Yeah, Mom, it's okay."

And she'll say, "You better put some ice on that."

I think my mom's attitude was, "We've got this issue. We want to err on the side of caution, but, at the same time, I don't want this to become a psychological impediment for my son as to what he can or cannot do." Certainly in the realm of physical activity there are limitations, but beyond that, anything is possible.

She always told all of us we could do or be anything we wanted.

I was born on Christmas, so people always say to me, "You must feel gypped. I mean, you get one present and you don't have a birthday."

And I say, "Well, I guess."

My mom would give me two presents and other people in the family would say Happy Birthday and then Merry Christmas. But I never had a birthday any other time, so how the heck would I know what it was like to have a birthday other than that? That was me. That's when my birthday was.

That's the way it's always been and I guess I treated the hemophilia the same way. It was part of me.

Did I go down to the park when I felt good and play ball with the kids whenever I got a chance? Yeah. Did I get whacked around and hurt and have to come home and take medicine? Yeah, but I tried to learn my limits. Sometimes I just couldn't resist it.

I was playing football in my own front yard when I broke my leg at age twelve. I was in the seventh grade, and I didn't break it by being tackled. It was

This photo was taken in June 2004 at Wendell's son, Cheo's, graduation from Weston High School, Weston, Massachusetts. They are, from left to right: Noni, now 24, who will finish her Master's Degree in English at Georgetown University this May (2007). She will be looking to work for a publishing company for a year or two before continuing on for her Ph.D.; Milele, now 34, is an OB/GYN physician in Atlanta. She and my son-in law, Alvin, a financial analyst, are the parents of the twins pictured with me on page 60. Next is Cheo, now 21, a junior at Connecticut College in New London, Connecticut, majoring in Theater and African-American Studies; and finally, Dara, now 29, who is currently living in Costa Rica, teaching English and working in environmental science. Dara will begin work on her Master's in Education at the University of Washington-Seattle in September 2007.

my mom calling us for dinner. I had to climb over a mound of snow or ice to go into the house, I slipped and fell and forced my leg beyond the range of motion and broke my femur. That was probably the worst injury I've ever had.

I went through the whole rehabilitation process for that injury, but apparently at that age and stage of my life, the injury affected the growth of my leg. They called it the "growth plate" in the femur, and as I grew larger and taller, my leg didn't. As a result, I had to wear a lift on my left shoe.

When people ask me "What happened to your leg?" I say, "Old sports injury."

I remember the pain. Pain was the hardest, but I think the pain made me stronger in some respects. In many cases, there was nothing I could do. I had to either live through this pain or — I don't know what. I would find different ways of getting through it, mostly by telling myself, "It can't last forever. It's going to get better. It's going to get better," and eventually it did.

I remember pain in all parts of my body, probably mostly my knees. That was the thing that was the most painful. I had other target joints, too. I have elbows that today won't straighten all the way out. I have a shoulder that gives me a little trouble now and then. I have an ankle on which I wear a plastic orthotic brace, rather than getting it fused. These are just things that I've gotten used to.

It's the pain and arthritic joint damage that causes certain limitations. For example, I can't ride a bike and, now, I don't even try. I have some difficulty going up and down stairs and I had to get a knee and a hip replacement about eight years ago at age forty-something.

I guess I'm thankful, first, to be able to have joint replacements; secondly, that my limitations aren't as bad as they could be. I can walk. I can go up and down stairs. I can drive. I can't walk too long without some discomfort, but, then, I hear other fifty-something-year-olds say the same thing!

I have a standing order for Tylenol, but I don't take much. I don't like pain medicine unless it's post-surgery or something extraordinary like that.

I want to feel how bad it gets and then I want to feel it getting better.

Pain puts you into a very close relationship with your body. You know how it feels and what it tells you, and I think I know my body pretty well. I can usually tell when something's coming on. I can tell probably within the first ten minutes what's going to turn into a bleed.

When cryoprecipitate came out, even though it was a frozen blood product, it significantly increased the potency and reduced the amount of medicine that had to be taken. That meant you could thaw it out and administer it much faster. I remember huge — they must have been 250-300 cc bags — of orange juice-colored plasma dripping in over three or four hours when I was a kid. With the cryoprecipitate, you have this little thin bag of clear liquid and, even now that I'm bigger and older, that's all that is required to produce the same effect that the large bags once did.

The antihemophilic factor and the home infusion — those had the biggest impact on my quality of life because they made access to medicine almost immediate. Within twenty minutes to a half hour, you're infusing.

In my lifetime, I went from four-hour visits to the emergency ward at Children's to twenty minutes at my counter in the kitchen taking care of myself. I can see how far the technology has come.

I was oblivious to the possibility of HIV because I was thinking, as I believe most of us were, that the factor we were taking was safe.

My recollection is of going in for a hemophilia check-up, being told that HIV was a concern and being asked to take the test. That was in conjunction with one of my wife's pregnancies. It came at the same time and then it was like, "Whoa," because naturally there were issues around the health and safety of my wife, Margo, the child and myself.

When they said, "Well, testing is something we're asking everybody to do," that was probably one of the scariest times.

I was totally convinced that it was just God's grace that I did not test positive — not that those who did test positive were any less deserving of the grace of God.

It was with a sigh of relief and a great deal of gratitude spiritually and otherwise that we learned that HIV was not part of our fate.

I could not have gotten through without my faith in my Lord and Savior. That's something I grew up with as a child. It is a very deep part of my being and that of my family. When it came right down to it, faith saw me through some of the periods of time when things were really, really dark.

If I hadn't had my faith to lean on, I don't know what would have happened. Maybe I would have snapped somewhere along the line or had a whole different attitude about life.

Sometimes, I would be lying in the hospital as a result of an injury, trying to recuperate from pain and wondering how much of my old self I'd get back. I would lie there in prayer saying, "Well, I don't know what this is all about, but I'm supposed to learn something; it's going to make me stronger in some respect and I'm just kind of excited to see how this all works out."

I have the battle scars of hemophilia in terms of joints and other limitations, but I missed the bullet called HIV. Wonderful. Now, on the other hand, a few years ago they told me I had hepatitis C. Okay, so HIV wasn't mine, but this is mine.

That's all right. We'll deal with that. It will be okay. It will work out.

When I met my wife, we were both in college. She was studying to be an RN and maybe she had a better understanding of my disease than someone else might have. It didn't seem to make any difference, at least not one that she ever talked about. Beyond concerns that I might have shown, I guess one thing that I liked about our relationship was that my hemophilia was never front and center with her.

I don't want anybody feeling sorry for me. I want people to see me for who I am in my head, not as a person with hemophilia. I don't want people to think, "That's Wendell, the hemophiliac, who is also a nice guy."

I've read stories in the *Hemophilia Magazine* about different challenges that families have had to face, for example, people living in rural areas where it's a three-hour drive to the nearest hospital. I understand that people can't choose where they're born, to whom they're born, their situations in life, what country they're born in, what race they're born to. You just don't get a choice. That's the way it is. I could have been somebody else, anywhere else, at any

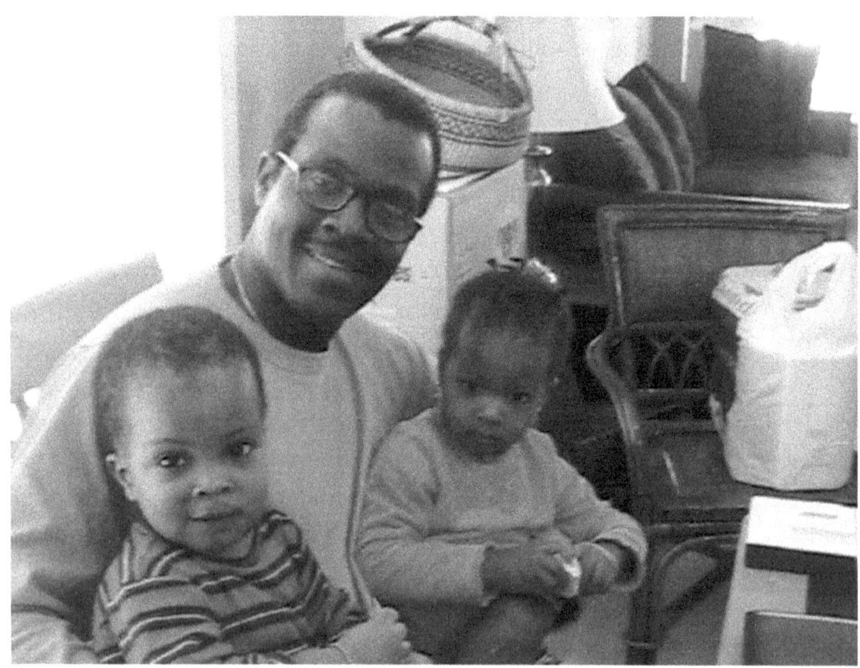

Wendell with his grandchildren, Eric and Arin.

time and that would have been the way it was. That would have been all right, but it just so happens that I'm me and I've had what I consider to be just a wonderful, blessed life and family under circumstances that have allowed me to deal with this the way that I have.

I think about that, and I'm very thankful.

My grandson, Eric, has hemophilia, and when he has grown up and I'm gone, I hope that he gets a chance to ask some questions about Grandpa and how he dealt with things. I hope that something I did helps him understand that you can just go ahead and do what you've got to do and live a life with God's help that is normal, just, good and in which you contribute.

You don't have to let this disease or anything else stop you.

"We've got a little something in common here, buddy," but my grandson's experience is going to be different because he was born into a different time. He doesn't have a clue right now, and it will be a while before he does. How he interfaces with his disease will be light years ahead of my experiences.

I had to learn to negotiate. I had tiffs and beefs with people: the macho thing on the basketball court or the playground, eying the same girl or whatever the case may be, but I self-developed negotiating skills, rather than the nose-to-nose, "Come on, come on, come on, I'll meet you outside." Things would rise to those levels, and I learned how to ease it down. I think that's why people sometimes, even now, see me as a peacemaker.

Parents could take a page from my mom's book around doing whatever they can to make their sons feel as normal as possible. Aside from the natural mother's love and the hugs and the way moms are with their kids, it is important not to put their sons in a situation where they wear this disease as some – pardon the expression – red badge of courage, in a way that clouds a clear vision of their goals and aspirations and ideas about what they can do in life.

I think my experience helped me understand people who are wheelchair-bound or have a disability. I understand when they say, "I don't want to be treated any differently than anybody else. This is who I am; this is where I

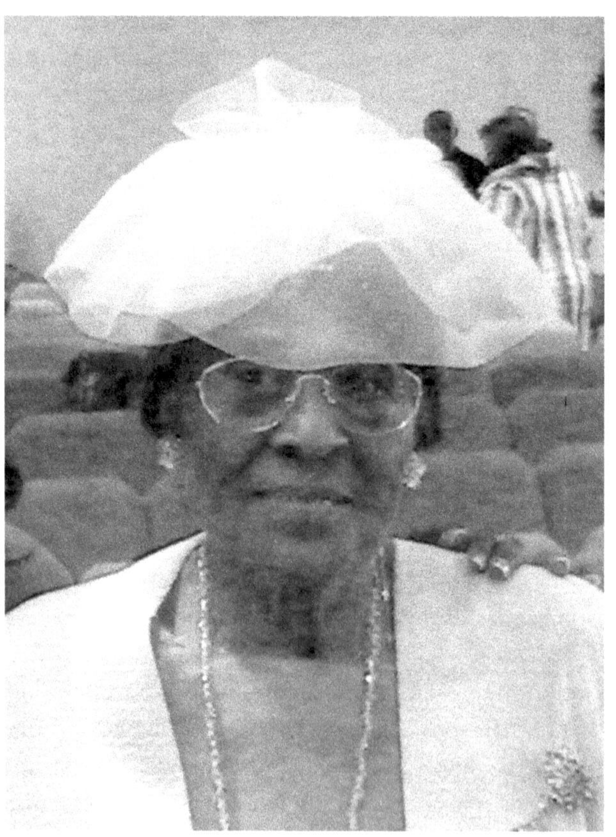

Wendell's mother, Abney Bourne.

am; but I can think, I can contribute, I can do."

So, no, I never did have resentment because, you know what? This was me.

There's never been another me. There's never been a Wendell Chester Bourne, Junior, without hemophilia, so I have no clue what it's like to be me without hemophilia. I just wouldn't be me then, would I?

On June 11, 2007, Wendell underwent a successful liver transplant at Massachusetts General Hospital in Boston. Six months later, Wendell wrote as follows:

"I can only say that I am grateful, first to God and to my family and friends and to the many wonderful doctors and other medical professionals who were involved with my case. I feel I was given a little additional time in life (none of us knows how long we have to begin with) to complete a mission, and I have promised myself and my God that I will not waste it. The liver transplant cured the Hep C-induced liver cancer and my hemophilia, but my 58 years of life experience as a hemophiliac will always define the lens through which I view life."

I came to understand that nobody has a right to claim God for themselves. God belongs to everybody, and every child we saw had a little bit of God in him.

Jocelyn Bessette Gorlin

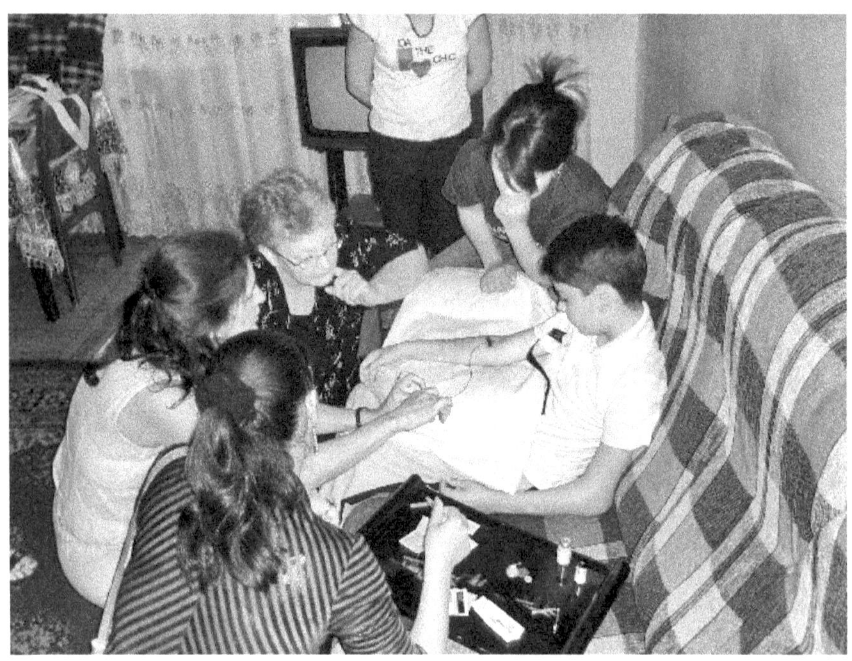

Jocelyn in Armenia with the World Federation Twinning Project.
(l to r) Jocelyn, giving the infusion; the interpreter; Margaret Hesiel-Kurth MD; mother, and child with hemophilia.

JOCELYN BESSETTE GORLIN

Mrs. Jocelyn Gorlin has been a pediatric nurse practitioner in hemophilia for more than 20 years. After obtaining her Master's degree in Nursing at Yale University in 1984, she moved to Boston with her husband and became the first nurse practitioner at The Boston Hemophilia Center. At the Center, she worked first with Diana Beardsley, MD; then with Bruce Ewenstein, MD; her husband Jed Gorlin, MD; and Ellis Neufield, MD. She has been active for several years in the National Hemophilia Foundation and the World Federation of Hemophilia.

In 1992 Jocelyn relocated to Minneapolis with her family, where she is now employed part time at The Children's Hospitals and Clinics of Minnesota Hemophilia and Thrombosis Center. There she is involved in clinical care, develops hemophilia nursing research and is involved with the World Federation Twinning Project. Jocelyn has had the pleasure of seeing hemophilia treatment change and improve throughout her lifetime.

I was lucky to have a great mom who was my friend as well as a wonderful role model. Our home was warm and welcoming, and she reached out to people, always willing to help. She wanted to be a nurse, but never was. Although my mother never encouraged me to become a nurse, I decided in high school that I wanted to be a nurse practitioner. As I look back, I think kids sit on their parents' shoulders, and I am proud to be sitting on her shoulders.

My husband and I moved to Boston from Connecticut in 1984, when I was only 25 years old. Jed was doing his internship and residency in pediatric hematology at Children's Hospital. There was an opening in hemophilia, and I applied for the position, even though I didn't know very much about the disease, nor did anyone really understand what a nurse practitioner was. I think they felt that I could learn about hemophilia, and as long as I was a nurse I would do just fine. Dr. Handin interviewed me, and he explained that he was starting a joint program with Children's Hospital and Brigham and Women's Hospital. He asked me how comfortable I felt working with AIDS, because they were starting to see AIDS with the hemophilia patients. I said it was OK, but I didn't really understand what it meant.

Around 1984, Diana Beardsley said to me – and I remember where I was sitting when she said this – that if you heat treat the factor it might kill the hepatitis and maybe even the AIDS virus. Many centers didn't want to switch to heat-treated factor because they thought it would affect the potency. We made a pledge that we would not use non-heat-treated factor, and we didn't. I remember writing "heat-treated" in big letters on an order for factor IX, and a person said to me, "You know, Jocelyn, we have a big stock of factor IX that's non-heat-treated, and I want you to use that." When I said no, I was told that I had to use it. I said no again, and I got into a lot of trouble. I knew that they wanted to get the non-heat-treated factor off their shelf, but I was not going to use it. And my husband, who is a doctor, said to me, "If you think that's the right thing to do, stick to your guns." And I did. I think we saved a lot of kids' lives because of that.

The program was initially called the Joint Comprehensive Hemophilia Center of Boston. I thought the name was too long, and suggested we change the name to the Boston Hemophilia Center. At first, Dr. Handin thought the name was too exclusive, but eventually agreed, and the Center was renamed. In the beginning there were only about 40 pediatric and 10 or 15 adult patients. Diana Beardsley eventually left to go to Yale and Bruce Ewenstein replaced her. Over time, we received more funding and hired Helen Mahoney-West, a wonderful nurse practitioner, and Cathy Cornell, a fantastic social worker.

We ended up taking care of 150 kids with hemophilia. I was told we were paged more often than anyone else in the hospital. It was really busy, and very different back then because there was no prophylaxis; I would say we saw between 5 and 11 kids a day. We saw so many bleeds, and every kind of bleed. Kids didn't have ports then, and sometimes we couldn't find a vein. I always told families that if I couldn't get it on the first two or three times, I would have someone else try. Occasionally, we'd have to call anesthesiology, and they'd come in to start an IV. Sometimes the kids would get stuck six or seven times. Can you imagine? We would stick one arm and then the other, and the arm would get puffy and the child would start to cry. The kids were really traumatized, but there was no choice. We had child life specialists and support groups and a social worker who would talk to some of the kids, but pain was a fact of life.

People now don't quite understand the pain that kids experienced back then. I remember Bobby Massie saying that having a bleed was like being in a house that was on fire. I also remember him telling me that one of the most important things for him was having his mom there, that even if there was pain, he still had his mom. And I used to say to all the families, I know this is very hard, I know, and I'm really sorry, but if you're there and you talk to your child while we're giving the factor, it will help. If you're at his head and you talk to him, he will remember that.

In 1985, AIDS started to show up, and they were putting bright pink signs above the kids' beds that said, "Blood and Body Fluid Precautions." These signs were hot pink, and it was heartbreaking because when kids with hemophilia were admitted, they slapped bright pink stickers on their chart and put them over the beds and on the doors. And the families would say to me, "Why are they doing this to us?" It felt like the Holocaust. Staff and visitors would put on gowns and masks when they entered the patients' rooms. They treated the kids with hemophilia very differently than the other patients. Speaking at one of the first AIDS conferences in Boston, I predicted that someday there would be universal precautions, where we would use gloves for all patients and not put signs above the beds. No one believed me. They said, "No way, Jocelyn, that is just never going to happen," but eventually it did.

It was like watching history unfold in front of your eyes. The association between hemophilia and AIDS had just come to our attention in the mid-eighties, but it wasn't well documented. There was a test called HTLV3, but we didn't know what a positive result meant. We knew there was an association with AIDS, but there was a thought at the time that the antibody might give some immunity to the disease, rather than be predictive of the disease. At the time, families didn't need to give permission for the test. We told them we wanted to test everyone for research purposes, and asked if they wanted to know the results. Some wanted to know; some didn't.

In New York City, patients were picketing the clinic, accusing the staff of knowingly giving factor that was infected with the HIV virus. We didn't experience this at our center. I think it was because Diana had switched to heat-treated factor so early and because Helen Mahoney-West and Bruce Ewenstein gave such caring HIV and hemophilia care. One mother who had a child with hemophilia was very angry with us when her child developed AIDS.

Nursing has turned out to be so many things that I never thought it would be. It has to do with health and physiology and psychology. It has to do with development, ethics and religion. We are supposed to take care of people physically, but it is really not about curing, it is about caring. I learned a lot in school, but I also learned so much from interacting with the families. As nurses, we are given a lens into people's lives that others don't normally have, and we are very fortunate. AIDS brought all this to a different level.

I was of childbearing age, and I knew that I could potentially get AIDS. I knew I couldn't get it from touching our patients, but I was drawing blood and I was giving infusions and we didn't have shields that protect the needles in the way they do now. Also, we didn't wear gloves. When I accidentally stuck myself one day, I didn't know who was positive and who wasn't. It was scary. There were a lot of feelings, of, you know, loving these kids, and yet being worried and frightened.

I took five years off to raise my children, and I came back to a whole different world. While I was away, factor prophylaxis started, and during that time, kids' lives changed. Before I left, I was telling them not to jump too high; now people were saying to me, "Jocelyn, they can run, they can play soccer." I laugh sometimes when I listen to myself talking with patients and families. I hear myself saying it's not okay to have a bleed. I don't want the kids to have any bleeds, whereas before children always had them because there was no prophylaxis. Now I tell them they have to take care of their joints because they are going to live to be 100. In the past, I could never tell kids that they would live to be 100, because they didn't. Hemophilia care has changed so much. Now they're going to have long-acting factor, and I think that will change lives even more.

A lot of people can't understand what people with hemophilia went through, or what the health care providers experienced. Caregivers who have been doing this for thirty years have unique stories that they carry around in their backpack and that becomes their own personal story. Only a health care provider who went through something similar can really understand. We have a bond. It is almost as though we went through a war together.

I know I don't know a lot about many things, but I know a lot about a little piece of history. All of a sudden, I realize that I have seen history. I have a historical perspective, and not all diseases offer that perspective the way hemophilia does, with so many complications and so many advances over a relatively short period of time.

I learned so much. One of the things I learned was how to be a good mom. I saw those mothers and they were great people. They fought for their kids. They were at school saying, "Let my kid do this. Damn it, I want my kid to do this." In their own quiet way, they were warriors. They were very strong people, struggling with something they hadn't asked for, but were learning a life lesson. These women showed me how to appreciate every day and how to pay attention. I learned to put things down when my kids sat on my lap and wanted attention. I know what to do when I am busy and someone says "Mom, I want to talk to you." Now I stop and sit down and try to be there for the people I love.

The families also taught me about religion. Once we were at a hemophilia camp run by the Catholic Archdiocese of New Hampshire. They conducted a mass at camp, and all the kids lined up to receive communion. One inner-city African-American boy with hemophilia hobbled up to the alter on his crutches. The priest turned to me and said, "Is he even Catholic?" I said, "Of course he is!" If he didn't deserve communion, who did? I came to understand that nobody has a right to claim God for themselves. God belongs to everybody and every child we saw had a little bit of God in him.

Every day, I am just so thankful to be alive. I have immense gratitude to the families for teaching me to be grateful for every day, and that what is important is to just love each other now.

I know that everything I have in life, I earned, and I feel good about it.

I didn't start out with a silver spoon in my mouth, like some people do. I know that I've done it the hard way. Nobody handed things to me, so I appreciate it much more.

I tell the kids, "Work for it. Work hard. You'll get there some day."

Chris Kucinski

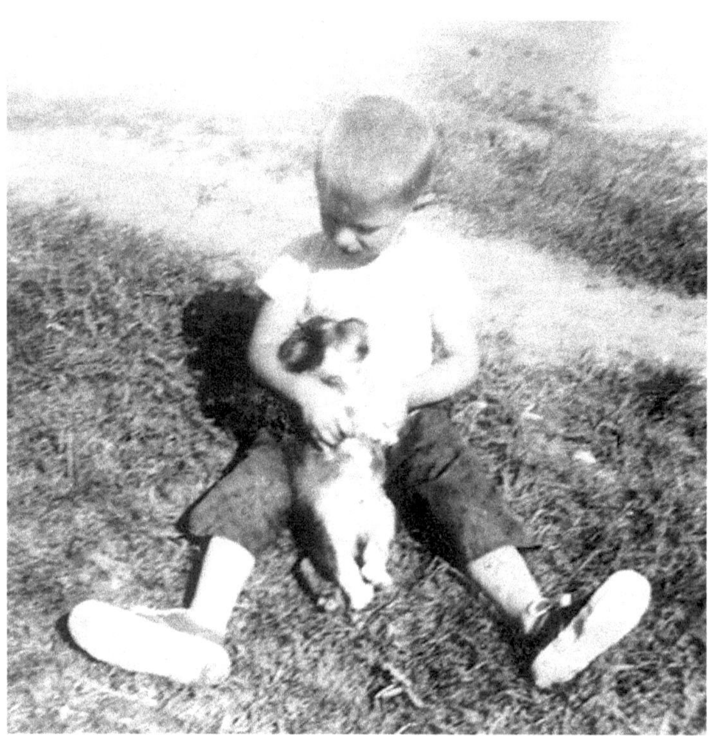

Chris Kucinski

CHRIS KUCINSKI

Mr. Christopher Kucinski was born in 1949 in Brockton, Massachusetts. Married, with five children, Chris grew up in a family of ten, seven of whom had hemophilia. Chris is loved deeply by his family and is a beacon of hard work and positive thinking. He has severe factor IX deficiency, HIV and hepatitis C.

I grew up in Brockton with my mother and father. There was a total of ten children in the family and my two sisters and one brother were the only ones who didn't have hemophilia, so there were seven boys in the family who had hemophilia. Junior and Bobby and Georgie died before I was born.

We lived in a big farmhouse and we worked hard in the fields, weeding, planting, picking vegetables. We had a farm stand out front and we built it up into a pretty good business. We all worked hard for my father.

My mother worked in a factory and did all the cooking for us.

When I got bleeds in joints and I couldn't straighten my leg or put pressure on it, I couldn't run, and sometimes I couldn't even walk. Sometimes I would hop on one foot to go to the bathroom or wherever, just to get around. I got real good at hopping on one foot. When I was real, real sore, my father used to put me on a chair, just a regular-type chair, tip it back and drag it on the two legs so I could go to the bathroom.

They say that hemophiliacs have what they call the "daredevil syndrome," that they try to do everything because they're told not to. You're going to have to watch any little kid who has hemophilia, because he's probably going to do the same thing we all tried to do, take risks.

Sometimes when you're young, you don't know what a risk is and what a risk isn't. Everybody else is doing it. Climb up the ladder. Go up there. Go do this. Jump off that thing. Then you hurt your leg and you don't know why you hurt your leg and all the other kids didn't. But that's part of hemophilia and part of understanding it.

Father wouldn't let us do much. He'd say, "Can't do this; you'll get hurt. Can't do that; you'll get hurt." We couldn't play or fight or do the stuff normal kids would do because they were afraid, but we used to horse around amongst ourselves and get hurt anyway. Dad thought if he kept us busy we'd stay out of trouble. That was his idea of how to help.

We had friends who came over, but we wouldn't usually go to friends' houses. Father just didn't want us to horse around and get hurt. When other kids came to our house, he'd say, "Take it easy with him. Don't bruise him up. They're bleeders. They bruise easy."

Oh, my parents were worried. They were always worried and concerned. Many times when I was at the hospital they said they didn't know if I was going to make it through the night. A priest came in and gave me last rites many times. I stayed in the hospital for thirty days at a time, minimum. Often, it was longer.

I didn't understand it at first, not when I was younger. I just couldn't understand why all of a sudden my leg would get stiff and swollen and I couldn't move it. I'd be outside trying to walk and I'd say, "I can't — what's the matter?" I just didn't understand why my leg wouldn't work, or why I'd get a bleed, or why all of a sudden, when I woke up in the morning, I couldn't step on my foot because it hurt.

And they would say, "You're a hemophiliac. It means you bleed in the joints."

I wasn't a doctor so how could I take that in and understand it?

We had home teachers. I went to school, but I couldn't walk. I couldn't take it. So a teacher came in five days a week, I think it was, for a couple of hours a day. I graduated from high school that way.

I was always smiling and happy. I always had a smile on my face and I was always joking around. I wasn't serious about things.

We had a lot of fun, me and my younger brothers. We horsed around, did everything together, the three of us, me, Jeffrey and Kevin. We hung out together.

In the winter we used to slide down the hill on sleds. We would get two hubcaps and we'd sit in one, put our feet in the other, then slide down the hill. We'd get hurt sometimes, but it was hard to keep us from doing stuff. When we were out of sight we did what we wanted. They couldn't watch us all the time.

I've always believed God's going to help me because I believe in God. I was taught that way — to believe. My grandmother told my mother, "Better to believe than not believe," and I asked my mother, "What do you think, is there anything to it?" She said, "It's better to believe than not believe," and I've always believed.

That was the right answer.

Am I going to sit and cry in my beer all day, or am I going to just carry on and do everything? I got married; I had kids. I raised plants and did some landscaping when I was younger. I worked with my other brother driving a truck and doing a few other things. I always tried to do as much physical stuff as possible. Even though my legs and joints were weak, I still kept going and trying to do whatever I could — just like anybody else. I mean, I knew I was limited, but I still tried to get around the limitations whenever I could.

As long as my hands were working, and they always worked better than my legs, I tried to do things — fix things, build things. I did a little carpentry work when I could. I used chainsaws and cut firewood. It was dangerous, but I'm very careful and try to get into a good position before I do anything, so that I don't take a chance of getting hurt.

When I went into the hospital on an emergency, usually my father was there to give a pint of blood to get me started. I would often have thirty pints of blood at a stay. I remember them doing quick cut-downs when they couldn't get a vein. They'd cut across my vein and then put a needle in. I had tiny veins and they had a problem with them all the time. I still have scars on my legs where they had to cut the veins open.

I had pain, oh, I'd moan and cry all night with a shoulder or a big knee, or an ankle that would swell up.

Once in a while, my mother would call the doctor and we'd get some codeine and that would help. It would knock you right out though. It was real strong. And that was a very hard drug to deal with. You wouldn't get it very often, only if you were in enough pain that it would make you practically cry. It was hard when we were in pain like that.

I can take a lot of pain before it makes me cry, before it makes me sad enough to break.

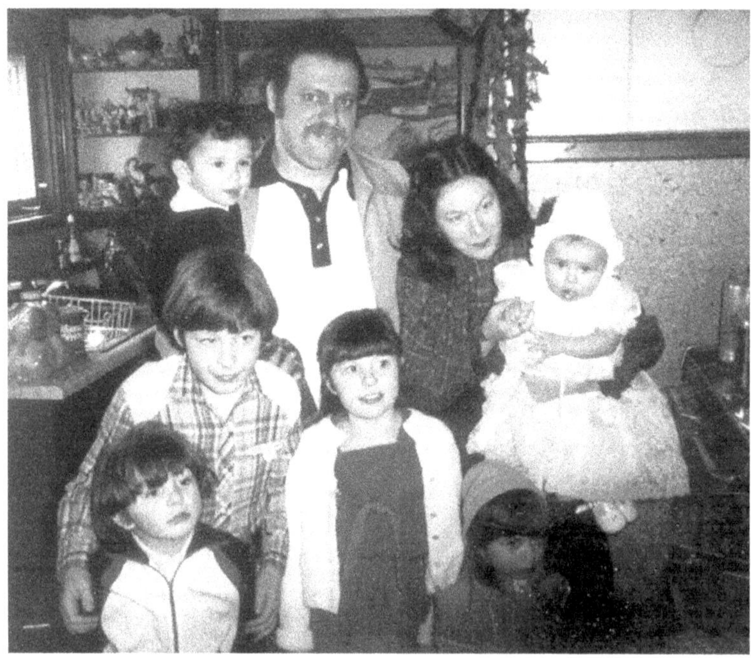

Chris (top center)

When you were in pain and injured, it was hard, but you didn't dwell on that. You tried to dwell on the better stuff, the good things, the things that you liked to do. We used to like eating. My father and mother both cooked and we'd have all homemade food: potato pancakes, French fries, American chop suey, Polish golabkies and pirogies. It was real good.

You could see in their eyes and in their faces that they were distressed, but my parents wouldn't let on that they were upset.

"What can I get you?" they'd say, or, "What do you want? Do you want some orange juice?" Want this?" "Want that?" Anything to try to help you.

"Want a wet face cloth? Want an ice pack?" They tried to do anything they could, but it was clear in their faces that they were suffering, too.

I think they handled it the way it had to be handled. If they had said more about it, then maybe we would have felt worse. It was probably better that they didn't say more.

Around 1969, we were told to go to Children's Hospital where they had factor. We met Dr. Sherwin Kevvie there, and he said, "We can help you."

With the factor, we didn't get as lame, as often. If we could get in at the start of a bleed, before it went into a full bleed, we could stop it. I'd go, oh, months at a time without a bleed with the factor. Months. I was able to do a lot more things with a lot more ease.

If I had had factor when I was young, I wouldn't have gone through half the things I went through. I'd have been treated quicker and healed up quicker and had a much easier life.

Bobby was twenty-three years old in 1962 and he was driving a tractor or something. Somehow, one of his kidneys started to bleed. He went to the hospital, but they couldn't stop the internal bleeding and he died.

Then I started thinking, 'How much time have I got left? What about me if something like that happened?' I always had that in my head. "Will I live to be twenty or thirty or forty?" I kept asking.

"I hope I live to such and such an age," then, when I reached that age, I'd say, "I hope I live to such and such an age," and like that. Bobby's death put the thought into my head that I was in a dangerous place.

I didn't tell most people that I had hemophilia. They wouldn't understand. They'd ask, "How come you limp? What's the matter with your leg?" and I'd say I hurt it this way or I hurt it that way. When we were kids, they would tease us and say, "Oh, bleeder. You're a bleeder; you're a hemophiliac." It wasn't nice.

My wife understood. I went over it with her before we were married and asked her if she was sure she wanted to go through life with me. "The problem is," I said to her, "that I can't take you out dancing. I can't do this. I can't do that."

"I'm going to tell you right up front," I said, "don't expect too much of me. There's a good chance that I'll have problems further down the road, too."

But my wife didn't mind. She didn't care. She understood. Every time I'm sick or every time there's been a problem, she's been right there. She was there every night in the hospital. I told her many nights to go home; I told her that she didn't have to visit me, to take a couple of days off, but she wouldn't do it. She's really been good.

The doctors and the Hemophilia Association said, "Oh, we're starting to hear that people are getting sick," but we didn't understand what HIV was. They said to keep taking the factor. They didn't worry about the risk of getting HIV because they didn't even know what the disease was or whether they could treat it or not.

In 1983, I got up with night sweats. I was HIV positive.

I started saying a lot more prayers then. I figured I only had a few years to live, based on all the stories going around about how people were dying. I started taking AZT around 1990. They kept checking my numbers and the numbers stayed in decent shape, so I started believing things were doing better. I've been saying lots more prayers since then than I ever did before.

Prayers to live, prayers to be healthy, prayers to stay with my family.

At first, people seemed to be prejudiced against anybody with HIV. If you told them, they blackballed you.

I thought the doctors were going to be afraid to touch me or shake hands, but they shook hands and intermingled just like anybody would. I thought they would put on rubber gloves and say, "You stand over there while I talk to you." I was afraid because they said that it was so contagious and so deadly that the health care workers wouldn't know what to do. I was afraid the doctors would shun me, but they weren't like that. People were always nice. They were always friendly, real professionals.

I know that everything I have in life, I earned, and I feel good about it. I didn't start out with a silver spoon in my mouth, like some people do. I know that I've done it the hard way. Nobody handed it to me, so I appreciate it much more.

I tell the kids, "Work for it. Work hard. You'll get there some day."

I was disappointed that the pharmaceutical companies knew the factor was bad and yet they kept pushing it and selling it and letting people use it. That should have stopped way back at the beginning. And the government didn't do its part either, but I didn't hold that against them.

I said, "This is the way of the world because big business always thinks of itself." They sell defective cars and people get killed in them, but the companies would rather hire their lawyers to fight the suit than to stop making the cars, because they're making so much money. That's the way it is.

It's just like a draw. Ten thousand people are born; one has this; one has that. That's what makes the world go 'round — different people. Why we're born blind, why we're born with different infirmities and illnesses; it's just the percentages and you happen to be one of the ones that was unlucky.

I'm sure we all wish we could go back to the beginning of our life and set it up the way we want to, but that's not possible, so we've just got to deal with it the way it is.

Some people deal with it better than others. That's the main difference.

What I think about death is it'll come to you eventually, but I'm not worried about it. I'm not afraid. The thing I'm most afraid of is that my family will miss me or I'll miss them. That's the only thing that kept me going when I was facing death a while ago. All I kept saying was, "I don't want to go anyplace. I want to be with my family and I know they want to be with me." That's why I don't want to leave.

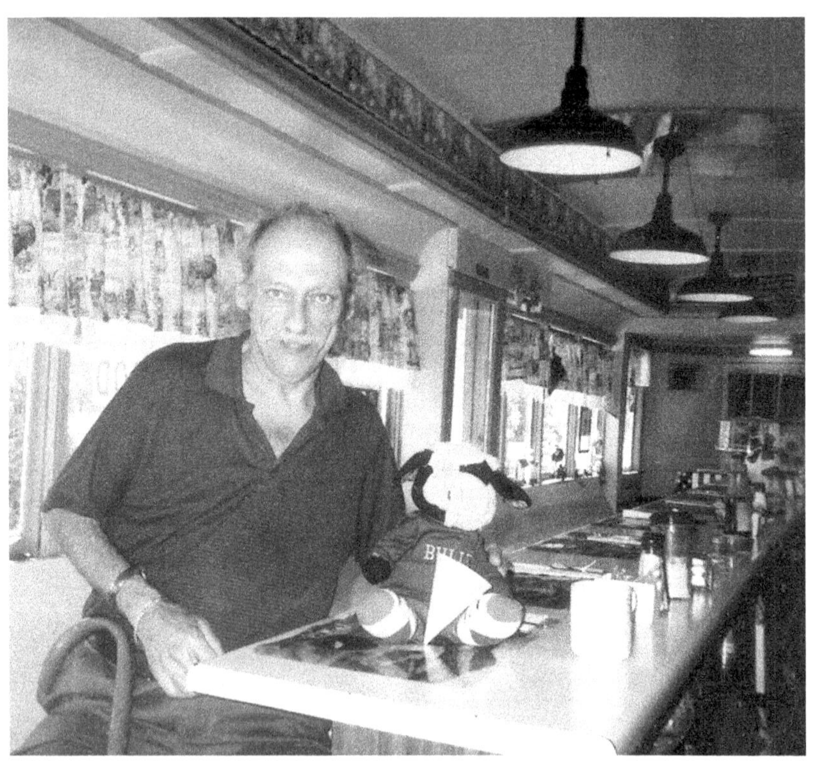

Chris

I don't think death is anything more than going to sleep and napping out. When that final time comes, I'll just close my eyes and be tired and go to sleep, something similar to that. I don't know what I'll see or what'll exist in my body and my mind and my soul, but I believe in God so, hopefully, there'll be a heaven for me.

Chris died in 2005

A ROYAL DISEASE*

Hemophilia has often been called the "Royal Disease." Queen Victoria of England (1837-1901) was a carrier of the hemophilia gene and subsequently passed the disease on to several royal families. Victoria's eighth child, Leopold, had hemophilia and suffered from frequent hemorrhages, which were reported in the *British Medical Journal* in 1868. Leopold died at the age of 31 of a brain hemorrhage. Leopold's daughter Alice was a carrier, and her son, Viscount Trematon, was born with hemophilia. He died in 1928 of a brain hemorrhage similar to the one that killed his grandfather.

Nicholas and Alexandra

Hemophilia played an important role in the Russian Royal family. Two of Queen Victoria's daughters, Alice and Beatrice, were carriers of hemophilia, and they passed the disease on to the Spanish, German, and Russian royal families. Alexandra, Queen Victoria's granddaughter, married Nicholas, the Tsar of Russia, in the early 20th century. Alexandra was a carrier, and her son, the heir, Alexei, was born with hemophilia. Nicholas and Alexandra were preoccupied with their son's health problems at a time when Russia was in turmoil. The monk Rasputin gained great influence in the Russian court, partly because he was the only one able to help the young Tsarevich. He used hypnosis to relieve Alexei's pain. The use of hypnosis not only relieved pain, but may have also helped slow or stop the boy's hemorrhages. The illness of the heir to the Russian throne, the strain it placed on the royal family, and the power wielded by the monk Rasputin were all factors leading to the Russian Revolution of 1917. In 1916, the 45-year old faith-healer Rasputin was assassinated in Petrograd by a group of noblemen bent on ridding Russia of the monk's corrupting influence on Nicholas II and Alexandra.

*Courtesy of the National Hemophilia Foundation, 2007

What offset the problems was the never-ending demonstration by my patients of their ability to respond to difficulties. This was a continuing blessing of the highest order and the greatest gift of all, not from me, but to me, from my patients.

Dr. Campbell McMillan

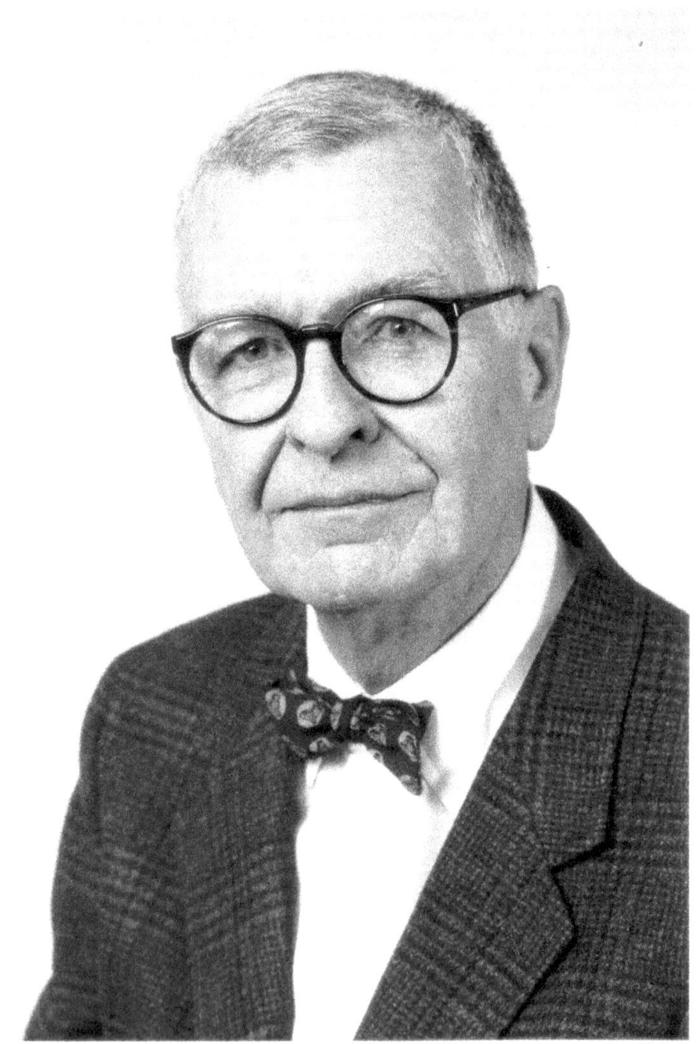

Dr. Campbell McMillan

DR. CAMPBELL MCMILLAN

Dr. Campbell McMillan's experience with the hemophilia community began as a pediatric hematology fellow at Children's Hospital in Boston from 1958 to 1961. Then, because of extenuating circumstances, he started a solo practice in general pediatrics in the small town of Laurinburg, North Carolina, from September 1961 to January 1963. At the end of that time, in response to an invitation to join the Department of Pediatrics at the University of North Carolina at Chapel Hill, he did so, becoming their first hematologist-oncologist. Until he retired in January of 1992, work with children and their parents in the hemophilia community was the principal focus of Dr. McMillan's clinical and academic activities.

In 1963 I joined the Department of Pediatrics at the University of North Carolina at Chapel Hill (hereafter UNC). During my years of professional care of children and their parents, I saw incredible changes take place; I really did. Fresh frozen plasma was the main form of treatment at the beginning, along with a few forms of factor VIII-containing fractions of limited usefulness. But far better things lay ahead.

Before coming to UNC, I had served as a hematology fellow with Dr. Louis K. Diamond at Children's Hospital in Boston from 1958 to 1961. Within the first few months of my fellowship, I launched headlong into the field of hemophilia, testing the agent which we called "Fraction One." This was the first commercially available fraction tested in hemophilic persons in the United States. It was truly a very primitive form of factor VIII treatment compared to what we have now. Drs. Diamond and Surgenor and I were the three authors of an article published in the *New England Journal of Medicine* in 1961 that described the effects of this early fraction.

The treatment we were using then was analogous to the short ride that Orville and Wilbur Wright had in their first airplane! It was that kind of thing. It was surely a far cry from the likes of recombinant factor VIII concentrates that we have now. But it was a part of the beginning and I was on the ground floor of the upward steps ahead. I am so grateful and proud to have been there! Also, those early days were vitally important to me in establishing the overriding importance of thorough and caring communication by physicians with children and their family members about treatment and all other concerns.

When I joined the department of pediatrics at UNC in 1963, I served all children with blood diseases, but hemophilia occupied a central focus of my work as a result of my fellowship training. In those days, the situation was far better for children with hemophilia, even with limited options for treatment, than it was for children with leukemia and other malignant diseases who were also under my care. Indeed, the initial discussion with the family of a child with newly diagnosed leukemia was preparation for the certain eventual death of this child. For children with hemophilia, the main problems were constant uncertainty and management of pain and the disabling effects of bleeding into joints and muscles.

In the early 1960s, there began to be important progress in the treatment of hemophilia. In 1964 cryoprecipitate from human plasma was discovered to be a significant concentrate of factor VIII. This finding was followed by development of factor VIII fractions in a variety of laboratories, including here at UNC in the program of Dr. Kenneth M. Brinkhous. By then, things were off and running in terms of improved treatment and the care that could go with it.

In the course of all these good things that were happening, what never left my mind was the host of problems that continued for children with hemophilia and their families. Foremost among these was the never-ending recurrence of pain from bleeding into their joints and frequent complications thereafter. On the other hand, what offset these problems was the never-ending demonstration by my patients of their ability to respond to difficulties. This was a continuing blessing of the highest order and the greatest gift of all, not from me, but to me, from my patients.

Then, in the early 1980s two major developments occurred with respect to the management of hemophilia: one was very good and the other was very bad. The good news came from Bonn, Germany, where Dr. Hans Brakmann discovered an exciting new approach to treating patients with factor VIII inhibitors. This approach consisted of administering high doses of factor VIII repetitively over an extended period of several months. Many of his patients benefited from this approach and the inhibitors were overwhelmed so that conventional factor VIII treatment could be resumed.

On the other hand, the unspeakably bad development in the early 1980s was the widespread emergence of profound failure of the immune system in patients with hemophilia. This, of course, was AIDS, i.e., Acquired Immune Deficiency Syndrome, caused by a virus, unwittingly transmitted to our patients by the very blood products that we were using to treat them. In 1984 the specific cause of AIDS was nailed down in two scientific publications and soon termed HIV for Human Immunodeficiency Virus.

And so, in those very dark days for patients with hemophilia and all persons involved in their care, a whole new dimension was upon us. The progress we had been enjoying was dreadfully dashed by the fact that the majority of our patients developed AIDS, notably more than half our patients with severe classic hemophilia. The death rate for affected patients was extremely high and remained so until assurance of safe treatment for persons with all forms of hemophilia was well underway by the late 1980s.

There is simply no way to capture adequately in words the fears that families and I faced together in treating their children who were either definitely infected with the AIDS virus or susceptible to it. It was particularly difficult in the mid-1980s, when the cause of AIDS was very clear but the safety of products we were using was not. Thus, if a child came in with a joint hemorrhage that would predictably respond to abundant resources in our pharmacy, what do you do? Until it became very, very clear that a given product was unsafe, the child and the parents and I would continue to treat and hope for the best.

Now let me tell you about one of my patients and his parents, who illustrate, at least in part, the dilemma I have stated and how we resolved it in his case. At the outset, I am glad to report that things turned out very well for him, in contrast to far too many other children who died.

In the beginning of 1984 the family and I began to discuss the feasibility of treating their young son according to the Brakmann program, described above as "good news in the early 1980s." Besides severe classic hemophilia, this boy had developed early in life a very strong and persistent factor VIII inhibitor and, as a result, had been essentially unable to enjoy any of the benefits of progress available to others without such inhibitors. On the other hand, even though he did not have AIDS at that time, evidence of this devastating disease was all around us and the safety of factor VIII products in high and sustained doses could not be assured, even with the best we had at that time.

In any case, in May of 1984, with our eyes wide open, the Brakmann program was instituted with no holds barred, and it worked out remarkably well. There was virtually complete suppression of my patient's inhibitor and he was able to resume conventional factor VIII therapy, which has continued into his present adulthood. Thereafter, he did develop AIDS, but it came at a time when effective anti-HIV treatment became available. He now shows no evidence of AIDS and responds well to factor VIII treatment, which he administers to himself.

How I wish there were more stories like his to tell about the children with hemophilia and their parents in the dark era before AIDS came under control. At the present time, through remarkable advances, safe products for treatment are flourishing. Indeed, the possibility of a genetic cure of some, if not all, forms of hemophilia is no longer an impossible dream.

I completely retired in 1992, and in my office at home the pictures on my walls include two treasures that are specifically relevant to what I have been saying. One of these is a leather-framed color print of a little boy in overalls and bare feet, sitting on the edge of an examining table in one of the rooms of our UNC pediatric screening clinic. He is holding his left foot with his right hand. His gaze is directed upward with his eyes showing hope and no hint of pain. His parents sent this picture to me a few years ago as a Christmas present. That little boy is the person I described above who underwent the Brakmann treatment program in 1984.

The other treasure in my office is a picture featuring a black and white hand-drawn likeness of a seated young man playing a guitar with his left knee crossed over his right. At the top of the picture his full name is shown and just underneath are his years of birth and death. He was one of my former patients with severe classic hemophilia who died of AIDS in the late 1980s. The rest of the picture contains a transcription of remarks at his funeral by one of his professors in the college where he was in his first year of graduate school in music. I would like to conclude my statement by quoting the last three paragraphs of his professor's remarks. I am using the name "Dave" for this young man instead of his real name to preserve his anonymity.

"Perhaps the quality that I will remember most about Dave was his love of life. That expression has become almost a cliché, but Dave gave it meaning. I can speak best about his attitude towards music. He did not merely listen to music, he soaked it up like a sponge – everything from rock and roll to jazz, Bach, and Mahler. One of my great pleasures was watching him react to recordings that I played in class. If he liked a piece, which was most of the time, he seemed to live every moment of it – the joy, sorrow, humor and passion. At such moments Dave gave me, without knowing it, a great gift: he reminded me why I chose to be a teacher.

"Dave was himself a teacher, although for only a short time in a formal sense. Nevertheless, he made an impact. In his first year of graduate school, he tutored students in music theory. Let me read from a letter that one of Dave's students wrote to me about him: 'Dave was what we would wish to be. He was never too busy to help me with my music, a subject in which I found myself way over my head. My grade of F became a C and then an A in a very short time. Dave was never too busy to care; day or night he was always available to me ... In the end, he was at least as satisfied by my accomplishments as I was myself.'

"I can think of no higher praise for a teacher than that. The last few times I was with Dave, he told me how much he had come to love Beethoven's music. Dave identified with Beethoven and other composers who had, as he himself had, struggled to live life to its fullest extent. I think that Dave understood their lives and his own in a way that I pray all of us may – as a free gift from God, but one given with a purpose. Whether consciously or not, Dave realized that purpose and used the gift of his life in a way that made those he loved and who loved him better persons. Dave can say with St. Paul: 'I have fought a good fight, I have finished my course, I have kept the faith.'"

To "Dave" and his professor and to all the persons with all kinds of hemophilia and to their families whom I have known over the years, I say "AMEN."

It was very painful and it was very embarrassing – very embarrassing. You know, when you're a kid you want to be able to be tough, and you want to be cool and there was nothing cool about this. Pain is awful, not just because of the physical pain and how that went untreated, but because it removes any ability you have to sort of keep a face on.

Dr. James Martinowsky

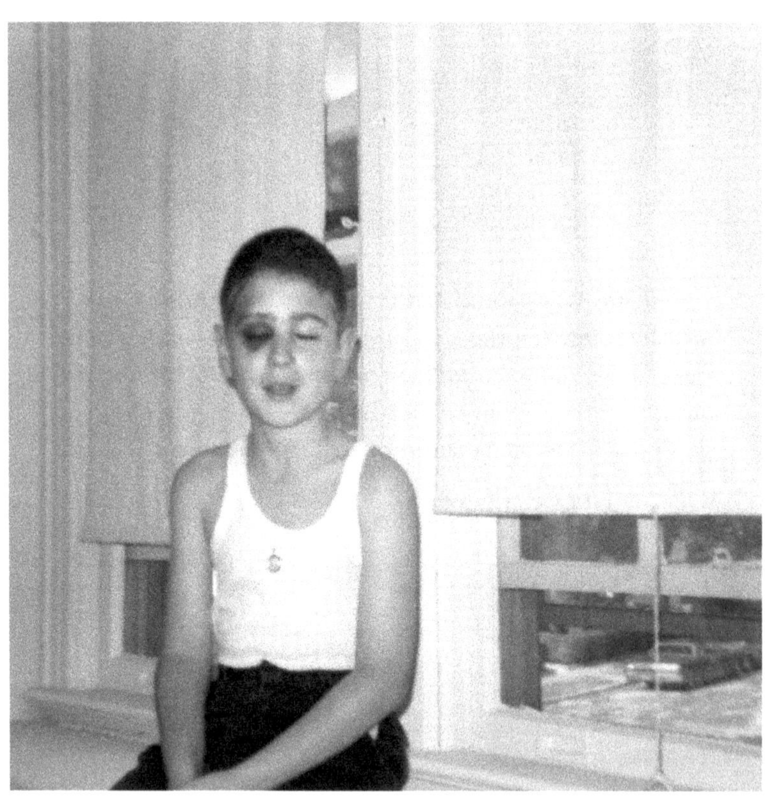

James, age 12, with a black eye resulting from the harmless toss of an acorn in his direction by his ten-year-old cousin.

DR. JAMES MARTINOWSKY

Dr. James Martinowsky was born in 1953 in Washington Heights, New York. He has moderate factor VIII deficiency and hepatitis C. He is married and has one teenage son. James teaches and practices as a child, adolescent and adult psychiatrist in the Boston area. He attended medical school in New York City, training and practicing on the same wards and clinics where he was treated for his hemophilia as a child. He believes the long-term psychological damage from hemophilia often outweighs the physical damage.

There was no family history. There were some suspicions. The assumption I grew up with was that I was a mutation.

My mother was really there for me. On the other hand, she wasn't actually always very assertive in terms of getting the best care for me. It was very hard for her. She was very intimidated by doctors, by medical people.

I think hemophilia was very painful for my father. I believe he couldn't face it, and it was not a problem related just to me. He was scared of the doctors and hospitals. Lots of times, we waited for hours and hours in the ER, and only as I got older would I start to speak up and say, "You know, you've got to get somebody down here to get the factor VIII." You know, to get the cryoprecipitate, or whatever it was.

It was also intimidating from a financial point of view. My parents couldn't really afford the product, and, although there was insurance, coverage could stop at any time.

It seems to me that I spent so much of my childhood trying to figure out when I would bleed and when I wouldn't, because it was so inconsistent.

I ate a pound of peanuts every day for a while. I found this letter that my mother sent to the scientist who'd written about peanuts, asking whether it was true that peanuts really helped with clotting. In his reply to her, the doctor said that, no, it turns out that they don't. But I still love peanuts, and I still sort of think they help me.

I have one memory of not being a hemophiliac. It was me being a very happy baby, with a wonderful disposition, just sitting there on the porch.

In those days, my mother and I used to refer to the hemophilia part of it simply as the 'bad old days'. They were referred to as the bad old days for how much pain was involved, for how much waiting was involved. It was an ordeal to get to the hospital and get treatment. It was a nightmare. It was three buses. Three buses each way.

It was very painful and it was very embarrassing – very embarrassing. You know, when you're a kid, you want to be able to be tough, and you want to be cool and there was nothing cool about this. Pain is awful, not just because of the physical pain and how untreated that went, but because it removes any ability you have to sort of keep a face on.

As a psychiatrist, one of the things I discovered when I was in practice was the importance of shame and embarrassment as emotions that get people into trouble.

My aunt and uncle used to blame me. They used to say, "How could you be doing this to your mother?" They couldn't understand why I'd gone out to play football or why I'd gone out to run. They'd think, "You know, how can you do that?" and they would yell at me.

I think my mother felt terrible about my hemophilia. I think she struggled with blaming herself. She once said, "It's all my fault." I started yelling at her that she could never, ever say that because it was my problem, not hers, and it meant that I couldn't ask her for the help I needed if she was busy blaming herself. It felt as though I would just be adding to her ordeal.

My hematologist was responsible for my taking charge of my illness. He used to speak with me, not with my mother. He cared about my psychological well-being. He really wanted me to have a sense of self and to learn about taking risks. He had seen people with hemophilia who had become so passive, who had become so fearful of getting hurt, that they had stopped taking chances.

By the time I was fifteen, I had become my own little expert on this illness and on medical things related to it.

I was fifteen. I knew what the bleed was about. I had been trying to dive, I had belly-whopped, I had started a bleed internally and I came pretty close to dying. I sort of lost consciousness. I heard them say that they didn't know whether I was going to make it. I had let the bleed go way too far, partly because I felt guilty about how I'd caused it. I'd been out with some friends trying to learn how to dive. I let it go on for a week of bleeding.

❧

The other thing that made one hospital admission different from any other admission was that two of my close friends visited me at the hospital. It meant that I wasn't so shut off. It was not the regressive experience that other hospitalizations had been. You know, my buddies came and we were hanging out there and I had choices all of a sudden about whether I was going to stay. That's the way it felt to me, at least. Other hospitalizations always felt very regressive. You felt like a kid. They're asking you for urine. You're being fed. You're being taken care of.

I remember screaming whenever I saw a needle. I had terrible veins and I remember they used to have me scream so that my jugular would pop and they could give me plasma through my jugular vein. They asked me to scream, and I liked that.

Access to veins was a very big problem for me. I'd go to the hospital and they'd stick me like sixteen times. The joke was that I was like a pin cushion, and it hurt. Your threshold for pain goes down and down, and by the tenth needle or so, the tenth time they're sticking you, you have no reserves at all, so it was just really agonizing. That was one of the reasons I was reluctant to go to the hospital.

❧

If they couldn't get access at all, they would send me home, and I was ready to go home. I was ready to bear another few nights of pain, whatever the joint was, and not be stuck over and over again. Sometimes, they would call their attending, and the doctors would be very frustrated about coming in. You'd have like lots of people enraged at you. I used to end up feeling just terrible about the whole thing.

❧

The character-disordered doctors would blame me for wiggling or blame me for screaming or blame me for moving once the needle was in. In fact, any time anybody got blood return, I froze.

Once the needle was in, I was so happy, thanking them and praising them. I would look for the same person the next time I was in the hospital, hoping that that person would be the one who would be drawing blood or putting a line in.

Once they got the line in, I would sit perfectly still for hours. The drops were slow because there was a lot of volume and they were always very worried about whether your body could take it. I would watch the plasma go in, this yellow fluid, drop by drop.

It was a blessed time when enough had dripped in and there'd be that moment when the pain would stop. The pounding, horrible pain would just stop and you knew that it was the beginning of the end of that bleed.

I think there is still a lot of ignorance today about treating pain. I used to hallucinate, I was in so much pain. I used to try anything. I tried to hypnotize myself into believing that I didn't have an arm.

"I don't have an arm," I would say over and over again, and then I didn't feel my arm, and I panicked.

One of the cruelest things about pain was that it really made me see things about myself that I could have better waited a long time to see, mind games, like what would I do to get rid of this pain? And you start wishing awful things on people.

I banned my mother from telling people, or interfering in any way at all. I absolutely wanted to be normal. I was more than willing to have a bleed and end up in the hospital, rather than be humiliated — or what I thought was humiliated.

My mother would scream at me to come back, yelling that I was going to get hurt, and then she'd start screaming at my friends.

"Don't go with him, Sheldon. Don't go. Don't play. He's going to be hurt; it's going to be your fault."

Sheldon will be at my son's Bar Mitzvah in about a month. My mother will be there. She's now in her eighties, and they'll joke about it.

Once in a while, my mother said "There are some things I'd rather not know," or something like that. She expressed that a few times when I was clearly going to be doing risky things and she clearly couldn't give me permission to do them. We had sort of an understanding.

My elementary school teacher met my brother on the subway some years ago and asked about me, fearfully. When my brother told her that I was a physician, right there on the subway, she started to cry. There was a belief held by some of the people who knew what was going on that I wasn't going to make it.

I think my sister was hit very hard by my having hemophilia. She was a year and a half younger and she was special because she was a girl, but I think that she really got less. I think it was very hard for her to ask for more of my mother's attention, given what was happening.

I'd like to think that when there are situations like this in families, if it doesn't break the family, it makes them stronger, and there are some data to support that.

When I worked on the pediatric ward of a rehabilitation hospital, I reviewed the literature on illness in families, and I think there are ways in which my family was fair and strong about things. There were ways in which my mother was seen as somebody who could be counted on, whereas my father, in his way, always stood by you. People master things, you know; people get through tough times.

I've done well. I didn't get HIV, you know, and all the other things that could have gone wrong. I've lived a charmed life, given how unlucky I was to have hemophilia; I'm an incredibly lucky guy. I still have a kind of magical thinking when bad things happen that it will be okay.

I felt that the medical system stunk. You know, I felt as though it was really patient unfriendly. I thought that it wasn't set up to provide efficient care. I thought that it was all about waiting. I waited in clinics for hours and hours all the time. I was waiting in a clinic at the hospital four hours to see a doctor who was just going to say, "Oh, your arm is better. You can go home now," or, "You don't have to come back for another three months." In fact, that's where I was, waiting for my name to finally be called, when the announcement came over the hospital loud speaker that President Kennedy had been assassinated. We were all in tears, then. That waiting stuff seemed to me incredibly wasteful and disrespectful towards patients and I don't think it's changed that much. Still a lot of waiting.

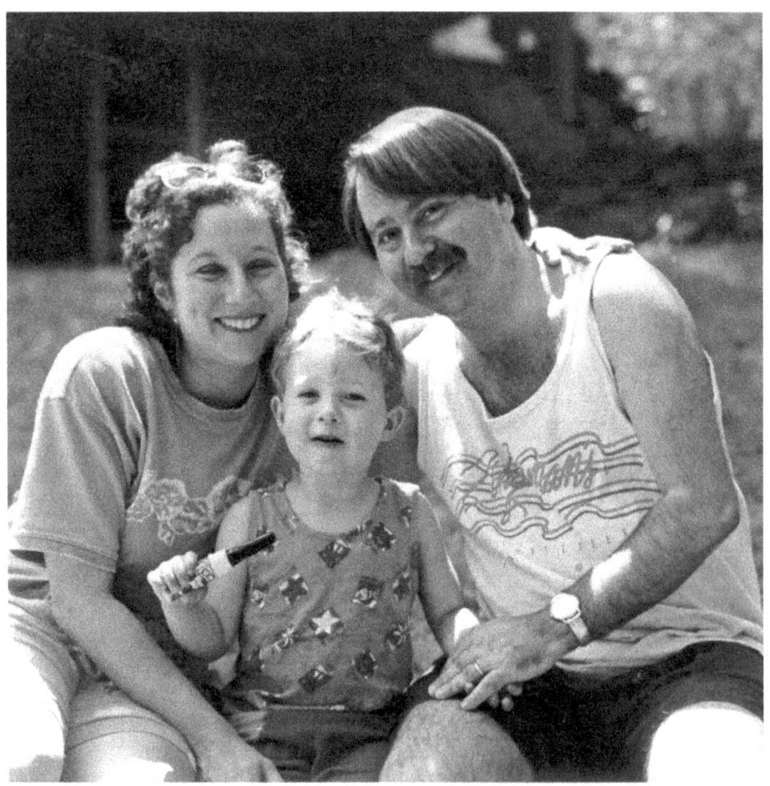

James with his wife and son in 1993.

If I had been asked years ago what my worst memory was of being sick, it would be babies crying, because when I was a little kid, they would always put me in with the babies. I was two or three or four or five, and all I remember are babies crying all the time while I was in the hospital. It was like this nightmarish sort of thing, crying babies in the hospital.

I used to rock when I was a kid, back and forth, a soothing activity and it also helped with pain. I rocked to the rhythm of the pain. It relaxed me a little bit. I remember they tied me down because I was rocking. They were afraid I was going to hurt myself.

What changed my life more was being able to travel with factor VIII concentrate. That was very cool. That was real freedom. I went to Europe by myself, just with factor VIII.

I had no question that I shouldn't have a child. I have hemophilia, okay, live with it, make the best of it, but don't give it to someone else on purpose. By the time factor VIII concentrate came out, it made a really big difference. It made me feel that maybe I would have children. With factor VIII, hemophilia was now more like a bother. It meant that I could be thinking about what I really wanted, which was to have a family.

My wife was actually very relieved when we had a son and not a daughter. She didn't feel great about the idea of having a daughter who was a carrier. It was something we discussed.

At the time the HIV concern arose, I asked if I could have heat-treated factor VIII and the director of the blood bank, my hematologist at the time, said that it would make factor cost twice as much money. I said it might work. He said there was nothing to worry about because the blood supply was not affected. I felt very, very angry at the way he dealt with it, and the way he dealt with it in an ongoing way.

I had gone to see Peter Levine once before for a consultation and I respected him a great deal. I thought highly of the idea of a comprehensive hemophilia center. Peter Levine had done it right and I really had a lot of respect for him and was very disappointed because he also felt that the blood supply wasn't infected. In his case, I think he just couldn't accept it. I think he loved a lot of his patients and I think he just couldn't accept that they were all going to be infected. That's my take on it.

It seems to me that hemophilia today is a different disease than the disease I had. Hopefully now, with the recombinant DNA, the risks are near zero, in terms of the horrible things like HIV. I think it's a different disease and it's great to think about that.

I applied to medical school in 1974, after factor VIII concentrate had been made available and the medical situation for hemophiliacs had changed dramatically, but it still was not easy. For example, I was told I could never consider psychiatry because a psychotic patient might strike me. I replied that I could probably give myself an infusion in plenty of time, since there is usually a delay in the onset of bleeding. I also explained that my approach, thus far successful, was to try not to let my illness limit me any more than was absolutely necessary. I was told that my denial was of concern and I was rejected.

Fortunately, I had very good grades and was accepted into a number of medical schools. I went to a medical school with an excellent reputation in New York City. It was a very difficult place for me to learn and begin to practice medicine. I worked on some of the same wards and clinics and with some of the same staff who had cared — and not cared — for me as a child/patient. Often, they had no idea, and it was very freaky when it came out. In the end, I think I only made it through all the post-traumatic stress symptoms (insomnia, nightmares, flashbacks, and brief moments of dissociation) by promising myself that as soon as I graduated, I would go into psychotherapy.

The reason I became a psychiatrist and not a hematologist was that in medical school it became very clear to me that the primary damage done to me was more psychological than physical.

Suffering is ultimately not good for the soul. You learn things from having been through a lot, but the price is much greater psychologically than whatever you gain.

Be active instead of passive in things — in choices. Make a lot of choices. Make mistakes.

I feel as though, yes, there is a God. Why? Because I've gotten through. That's the proof. I have personal faith that there is a God, and you know, since I was raised Jewish, I assume he might as well be that God.

I wonder a lot about how this experience will be passed on to my son. I wonder at times whether I say too much and at other times whether I say too little about it. I like the idea that there's this record. Maybe he'll want to know more. Maybe he won't. I'm not sure. It's a very special thing to have a healthy son.

I so believe that in each and every encounter as a caregiver, you do the most you can for each individual. That's the important thing for me, to know that I did everything I could possibly do each time.

Helen Mahoney-West

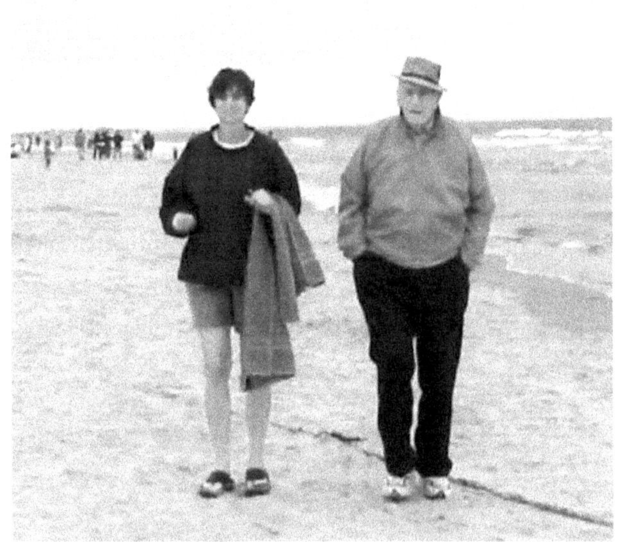

Helen and her father.

HELEN MAHONEY-WEST

While working as a Nursing Assistant at the Shriners Burn Hospital in Boston, Helen Mahoney-West attended Boston University School of Nursing, graduating in 1983. After taking her Master's degree in Nursing at Yale, Helen joined Dr. Diana Beardsley at the Yale-New Haven Hospital Hemophilia Center.

In 1990, Helen joined Dr. Bruce Ewenstein and the team at the Boston Hemophilia Center as the Hemophilia/AIDS Nurse Coordinator. In 2003, she moved to Children's Hospital in Boston as Nurse Practitioner, working with high-risk, HIV-infected adolescents.

Helen is currently on the full-time faculty at the Regis College School of Nursing.

I am one of eight children, and my youngest brother was born with very severe cerebral palsy. He only survived to be eight years old and he never walked or talked, so he was a full-care individual. Having him as my sibling led to my interest in nursing in the chronic care arena.

Because I could understand the impact of chronic illness on a family, I was always interested in the ring of influences that are present when you have someone you care about who is chronically ill. I think frequently about my mom and dad and the challenge of having eight children, with the youngest being severely disabled. I think about spreading yourself thin when you are taking care of someone with severe and chronic disabilities, because taking care of my brother took a real toll on my mother. Although she'll say she had a wonderful life, it was a hard life and I'm not sure how much that was recognized.

I know she thinks about it and I know she realizes that she really did something pretty remarkable.

My father, who was a college librarian, played a huge part in caring for the family and making sure people were taken care of. I feel strongly that my interest in people really came from my father, and the combination of my parents' strengths is probably what shaped me in terms of my interest in people and the path my life has taken.

When I first went to Shriners and worked with burn patients, I loved working with children and I also really liked my nursing experience. It was satisfying and it felt right. One came to see the disfigurement without it being shocking or unusual. I had my brother's example in front of me, and I think the most important thing was realizing that there was a big personality in him. He was a really sweet child, and the same thing was true with the burns patients. I knew that inwardly there was a person there who was really interesting; there was a person to whom I could reach out.

After earning my Master's degree as a nurse practitioner, I joined Dr. Diana Beardsley, who works with the hemophilia population at Yale-New Haven Hospital. I was interested in the position there because it involved pediatric chronic illness. By that time, too, it had become known that people who had had blood transfusions or who had received blood products were at risk for HIV, and I was interested in that work, as well.

We started to test people who had not been tested for HIV, because it was clear that everyone who had received blood or blood products from the late '70s through the early '80s was at risk for HIV.

I remember a couple of cases in particular. One was a very handsome young man, about eighteen years old, with mild to moderate hemophilia, who only came into the clinic once or twice a year because he did not have a lot of problems with bleeding. He was young, he was healthy, he was headed to college; he had professional aspirations, he was a good student, he was an athlete. He had had infusions of factor during the late '70s and early 80's, and even though he had not had many infusions, he was HIV positive.

I remember giving that information to him and to his family, who were very much part of his life, and how he tried very hard to accept the news and work through what it meant for him. It was really hard, but he tried to understand the diagnosis, tried to figure out what he had to do, but also live his life.

His mother was devastated. Time and time again, the mothers really carried the affect for the kids and for the family; they showed the emotion and the sadness, the anxiety and the fear. We would really pick that up in them.

The patients I worked with at Shriners Burn Hospital and the hemophilia population I came to know in New Haven and at the Boston Hemophilia Center in 1990, are very special people. Somehow they have been given something — some new insights — from their experience, and they come to value life in a different way. There is a greater valuing of each day and of the individuals they love and feel close to. I think that the relationships they have are frequently more loving and positive. They also know that there is more to life than playing sports, doing well, excelling; they know that the value lies more in the way they feel about things and in the way they relate to people.

The disappointments for these patients are often harder than for other young people. I think it is very difficult for those who have gone through a lot of trauma to cope with more, and sometimes the little disappointments become big. But in the end, people who have gone through a lot are usually able to go beyond the disappointments — and they have to, over and over and over again.

I believe that patients who can frame life in such a way that they see something good, either day-to-day or in a positive way overall, seem to do a little bit better than people who become bitter and depressed and angry. Some of the patients I worked with committed suicide because the changes that took place for them were so devastating. Some people become self-destructive; some people become drug-dependent and alcoholic in treating the depression and disappointment.

The true survivors have a couple of things going for them, and one of those is that they have some kind of emotional support. Frequently, in the hemophilia community, the family was key in terms of acceptance. The love, the encouragement, the support, the friendship, the companionship they received made all the difference. You do better when there is somebody helping you through.

It was much harder for patients who didn't have those resources, harder for them to continue to go through the disappointments.

The mind is very powerful. If you are able to conceptualize things that bring you joy and remember the experiences — things such as a relationship or a conversation or a place you love to be — that's really important.

That experiential knowledge is important. It makes a difference to have had some positive experiences from which to draw. If you've been able to go to a beach on a beautiful, sunny day and that occasion brought you joy, you always have that. You can always go back to that beach.

If you've been able to walk through a park or a garden when it was absolutely beautiful with someone who means something to you, someone who provided you with those experiences, that's key. If you've grown up in a family where there's love and friendship and if you've found pleasure from interactions and the playing that you've done, that's key.

When those things are missing, then it's hard.

I so believe that in each and every encounter as a caregiver, you do the most you can for each individual. That's the important thing for me, to know that I did everything I could possibly do each time. Then, in some encounters, there is not a lot for you to do and you have to accept that for some people you can do more than you can for others.

We had a really good team of people and that was essential. You have to be able to plan and process some of what is going on in your work with other professionals. Having good people to work with, colleagues with whom you can share the impact of any particular situation — when somebody unexpectedly gets very sick, or somebody you are very connected with dies — is really important.

At one point, we started having memorial services at the Hemophilia Center, and it was very helpful to have a quiet, special time. The little chapel was beautiful and we would invite families to share a real acknowledgement of the individuals who had died. A lot of healing went on in the preparation of that.

Being able to recognize a loss that you are all immersed in is part of life. Feeling as though you've done something to acknowledge loss is very important.

Most people working with hemophilia patients didn't expect to be dealing with HIV on top of everything else. There were nurses who found it really exhausting to work with patients for many years, only to have them re-diagnosed with HIV. That was very hard. Integrating the HIV and the AIDS into the hemophilia care became another challenge: some people were interested and some people were not. The task for a while was huge in terms of how to shape the care and how to think about it.

I mean, who knew? Nobody knew. HIV is not a good diagnosis now, when we have some hopeful treatment plans and long-term survivors.

At that time, it felt hopeless.

I am frustrated when I see people trying to deliver care quickly: when they're focusing on the billing, making sure they've got their numbers, making sure they're reimbursed. It is very difficult for me when systems are driven more by the bottom line than by patient care.

I believe that a lot of caregivers don't understand the power they have. When a patient comes to them with a problem — and it may be just an earache — something more critical than the earache is often going on. That patient may have no one else to go to who can understand and help him or her, and sometimes the caregiver doesn't take enough time to figure that out. The patient may be hungry and we don't take the time to give them a food voucher; that's what upsets me. That's hard for me.

Some nursing and social worker colleagues do understand the depth of the issues that patients face. A lot of the issues are very abstract, and the key is to try to help caregivers understand what it's like for somebody who has a young child that they have to bring into the hospital every month because of a bleed. When you understand that, then you also understand that those patients have lives that are hard and challenging.

That understanding is intertwined with your own personal and family life and the things you're trying to balance and juggle in your own world. I think the people who have had more experiences themselves will listen better.

I think about the richness of the families I have worked with and I will carry that experience with me always. I really loved the families; I loved the patients. I have so many of them in my heart. I derive personal richness from the work, and that's how it has affected me.

As hard as it is and as sad as it is, there is a real connection there for me.

And I said, "I need to do this. I can't just bury my head in the sand anymore. People need to know the truth," and that was the end of it.

Roy Arruda

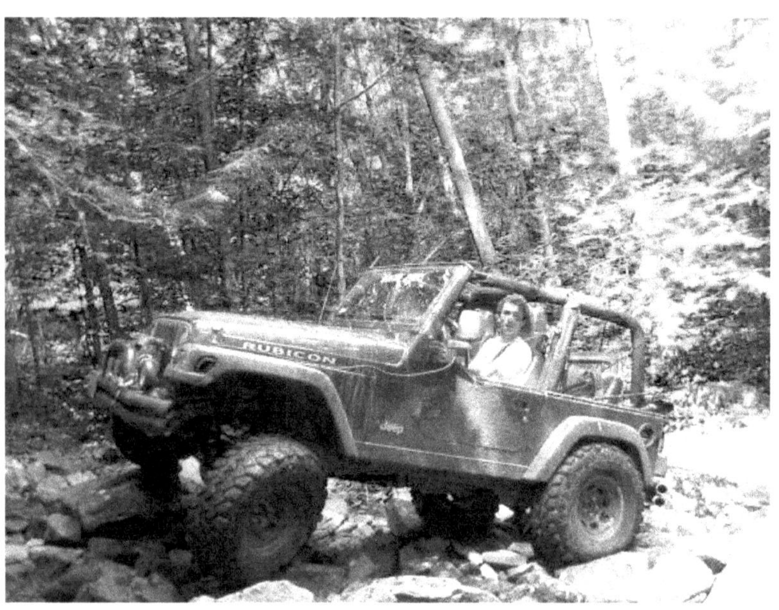

Roy at his favorite outdoor pastime: 4-wheeling in his Jeep.

ROY ARRUDA

Mr. Roy Arruda was born in 1960 in the Azores. His older brother, who also had hemophilia, died of complications from AIDS in 1995. Roy, who is not married, works as a nursing assistant with people who have AIDS. He is an avid hiker on the Appalachian Trail and a recreational all-terrain vehicle driver. Roy often speaks publicly about his and his family's experience in coping with AIDS. He has severe factor VIII deficiency, HIV and hepatitis C.

When I was six months old, I fell out of the baby carriage and cut my lip and my parents couldn't stop the bleeding. They took me to the doctor and that's when he diagnosed my hemophilia. Hemophilia is not something they looked for in those days in the Azores, where I lived.

The Portuguese doctor who diagnosed my disease, Dr. DeLima, said it would probably be best to let me die the next time I had a bleed. There were just not the resources on the island. In the Azores, we had to bring our own blood donor with us, because the hospital couldn't or wouldn't provide one. I had to bring my blood supply in on foot.

"This is not considered an emergency," the doctor said. "It's not a life and death situation."

But it was.

My father graduated from technical school and my mother finished third grade, which is the equivalent of a complete grammar school education in the Azores. It was really her decision to come to America. My father was hesitant because it was a big move and we had a house, extended family and jobs in the Azores. We had everything there, really. My parents knew that there were two countries where they could go. One was Russia, which had factor products, the other was the United States. We didn't want to go to Russia, so my parents decided that my mother and I would come to the United States for treatment.

I was twelve. My left knee was history by this time and my joints were deteriorating big time.

We didn't go back to the Azores. My mother said that she was staying here, in America. "This is best for him." My brother also had hemophilia, but his wasn't as severe as mine was at the beginning. He played whatever sport he wanted; he never got a bleed. My father sold the house in the Azores, the car, some land and he and my brother came over. We found an apartment. My father got a job, and we started from scratch.

My mother is a very determined person, a little more so than my father. My father tends to say, "Well, let's think about it." My mother says, "No, let's go."

I am very lucky that she is that way. It made all the difference in my care.

My father worked at a boat yard here, although he didn't know much about boats. You also have to remember that he didn't speak English, so he had to get a job wherever they would take him. It wasn't a great job, but something to help pay the bills. He didn't make a lot of money, but it did give him health insurance, which was crucial.

That's another nightmare, because every chance the insurance company got to refuse payment, it would. Cryoprecipitates weren't cheap and I averaged three days every other week in the hospital for a year or so.

That's expensive.

Every two weeks, I was in the hospital for two or three days. I'd get out of the hospital, spend a few days at home, then go to school, but I was lost because I didn't have a clue what they'd done for the past week. It was three years before I was comfortable with the English language, before I learned to speak, to write and to communicate.

None of us spoke English when we came to America. We had a friend who spoke both languages and we took her with us when we went to the doctor. Also, none of us drove. My father drove in the Azores, but we didn't have a car here. To have a license, you had to go to driving school, start from the beginning.

Our friend's husband worked in construction in Boston, and sometimes he would drive us in. We would leave at seven in the morning for a two o'clock appointment. They have a little garden with fountains at Children's Hospital and we'd sit there and eat breakfast and lunch while we waited for the appointment at two.

Dr. Manson and the people who worked at Children's provided me with a second life. I almost owe my life to them, you know, to the people in Boston, and I mean everybody: doctors, social workers, nurses, secretaries. Dr. Manson was the first contact there that I remember. He told us about the disease in more detail. He told us that I could live a normal life, do whatever I wanted to do.

Maybe I would never be a football or a hockey player, but that's the way it is.

I was beginning to have thoughts about what I wanted to do with my life. I was developing goals. It was a childhood dream to work with planes, and I was determined to continue on through school and work with jet engines. I wanted to build things or design things or fly.

Throughout high school, I was determined to live with the disease and put it on the back burner. I did not want the disease to control my life.

The first year of high school, I almost flunked out, to be honest with you, but I was determined that I would overcome this and I did. I managed to graduate from high school with a B+ average. I was determined to continue, because I wanted to go to college.

One of the problems I faced was that I couldn't come home and ask my parents for help with schoolwork. My parents didn't know how to read English. If you can't read, you can't do math. You can't do science. You can't do history. You can't do grammar. You can't do spelling. You can't do anything. So I had to depend on myself, I had to teach myself how to do things. I used a tape recorder to record the questions, then I would play it back and answer them. It was a little process, but it worked.

The information I had about HIV initially was from the newspaper and television; secondary information was coming from Boston Children's Hospital to my brother and me because most of the time we had appointments together. There were regular checkups, sometimes every three months, sometimes every six months.

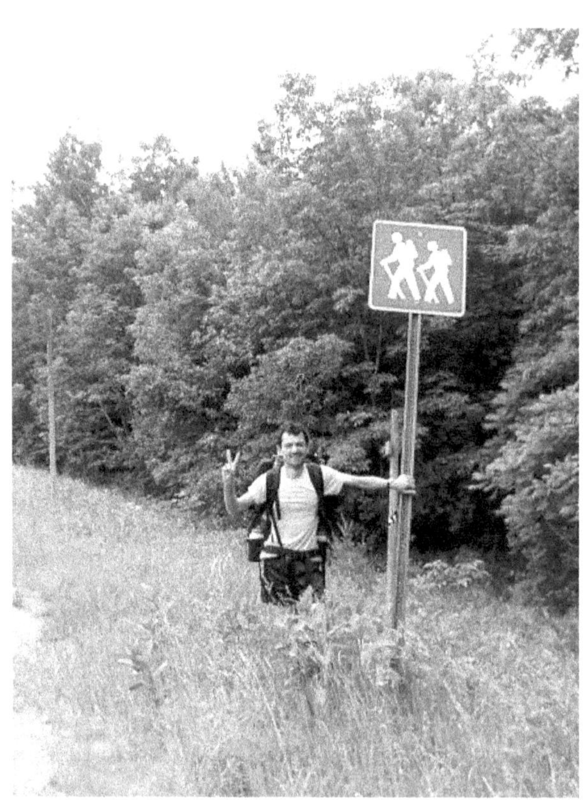

Roy hiking on the Appalachian Trail.

We sat, the doctor sat and he told us that our blood count was going down.

"Yeah," I said, "but I don't do drugs."

"Well, but you know, it's the same with people who are homosexuals."

I said, "Well, doc, I don't do that either."

He said, "Well—"

It used to drive me nuts. The way it was presented to us, my brother and me, was that it's a homosexual problem and an IV drug user's problem.

"Okay, so I don't do either one of those things and you're telling me that my blood count is dropping? What happened?"

"Well," he said, "we don't know what's going on. Maybe it's in the blood. We don't know what's going on."

At first it didn't bother me. I said to myself, "I'm not going to worry about this," but I was in rough shape. They were drilling it through our heads, "Your blood counts are dropping." My brother and I would come home and cry our guts out. That's how we dealt with it for about a year.

Eventually, they did say that most likely we had been infected through blood pro-ducts, factor VIII. They tested my brother. He was HIV positive. It was official. We knew. Every time we went up to the hospital, our blood count would drop two hundred, another two hundred, another hundred, so we knew there was a problem.

For the longest time, our parents said, "Oh, it will get better. Someone will come up with a cure, or a pill or a shot or something. Something will happen." We didn't look sick, my brother and I, so they believed it would be okay.

We didn't know any hemophiliacs who were really sick at that time. It wasn't until many years later that we finally knew that some hemophiliacs had died, and we said to ourselves, "You know, this is not good."

The people in Boston were very supportive. They encouraged me to continue to live a good life, as far as good nutrition and exercise, and if I was sexually active, they told me to use proper protection. They drilled that into my head every time I went up there. I suppose that's part of being a medical person.

I was not going to be a "man with hemophilia." I'd just be a man, period. After grammar school, I didn't want people telling me not to play this, not to do that or "Gee, is that contagious?" I didn't want to deal with it. I didn't want to deal with the politics. We definitely never told anyone about the HIV stuff. We just kept to ourselves.

In our family, we support each other. When we have a problem, we talk it over and resolve it within the family. We didn't go outside the family, particularly with the HIV stuff, because we didn't want other people to know about it. We are very close and we worked it out with each other. If we were too stressed, we'd just sit back and cry for whatever time it took us to get rid of the stress, then we went out and did whatever we needed to do. That was our way of dealing with the depression and anxiety.

Looking back, I wish we had done things differently, but I don't dwell on it.

There was a fourteen-year-old boy in Swansea, not far from here, who had HIV and the other parents took their kids out of junior high because they didn't want their sons and daughters to be in the same classroom with him. That's what it was like then.

My brother graduated with a degree in mechanical engineering from Southeastern Massachusetts University, the same place that I went, and he went to work for a company in Newport, Rhode Island that made parts for missiles. My brother was a go-getter. He wanted to be like everybody else. He wanted to be normal. He wanted to be able to talk comfortably about everything. He had to be around people. He couldn't be alone, totally different than I am. Somehow the company found out about his HIV status and pretty much after that he lost the job.

My brother, Joe, was thirty-one years old when he died in 1995, three years after he lost his job.

One Saturday, we got a call from the doctor to say that they had had to put Joe back on the respirator; he wasn't doing well. We went back up to the hospital and there he was on the respirator again, just lying there. Things were bad. His kidneys had completely shut down. He had a DNR, Do Not Resuscitate, and I was his medical agent. I don't think my mother would have been able to make the decisions I had to make at that point.

"Just keep him comfortable," I said, "and we'll take it from there."

"That's fine," the doctor said. He told me he didn't think Joe would make it. I was trying to feed my parents this information, but they didn't want to listen. They were in big-time denial. I told my sister, and she cried, but she accepted it.

The doctor called at ten o'clock at night and said, "You need to come down, Joe's having heart palpitations."

I went down and we were there when he died. That was in May of '95. That was the end of it.

My brother's death was like the icing on the cake for me, and at that point I said, "There's no way in the world I'm going to look the other way and stick my head in the sand." I wasn't sure what I was going to do, but I wasn't going to ignore it. I knew I was going to figure out a way to tell people about the stresses, about different ways to be exposed to HIV or AIDS. I wanted them to know how it had been for us growing up, the way the public treated us. My brother's death pushed me into that decision.

I told a few close friends – the social worker, the psychologist, the nurses.

"The wheels are turning," I said. "There's nothing to stop me now," and everybody warned me, "Slow down, Roy, slow down. You're doing too much."

"No, I'm not," I'd say. "I'm not done. This is just the beginning. You haven't seen anything yet."

I came home, sat down at my desk and wrote my life story. I wrote and wrote and wrote and wrote. I put together my life story from the beginning in the Azores to coming to the States and being treated at the hospital and going to school. Mostly I concentrated on the time when I was working and the different stories I'd heard. Then I told the people at the Rhode Island Hospital that I would present my story to whoever wanted to listen.

The people from Rhode Island Hospital were my guinea pigs. I presented my story there on World AIDS Day, December 1st, 1995, six months after my brother died. It wasn't too bad. I got a little choked up halfway through, but I did okay under the circumstances. My parents weren't happy at first, but then they said, "Okay, fine. I wish you wouldn't do it, but if you want to do it, go ahead."

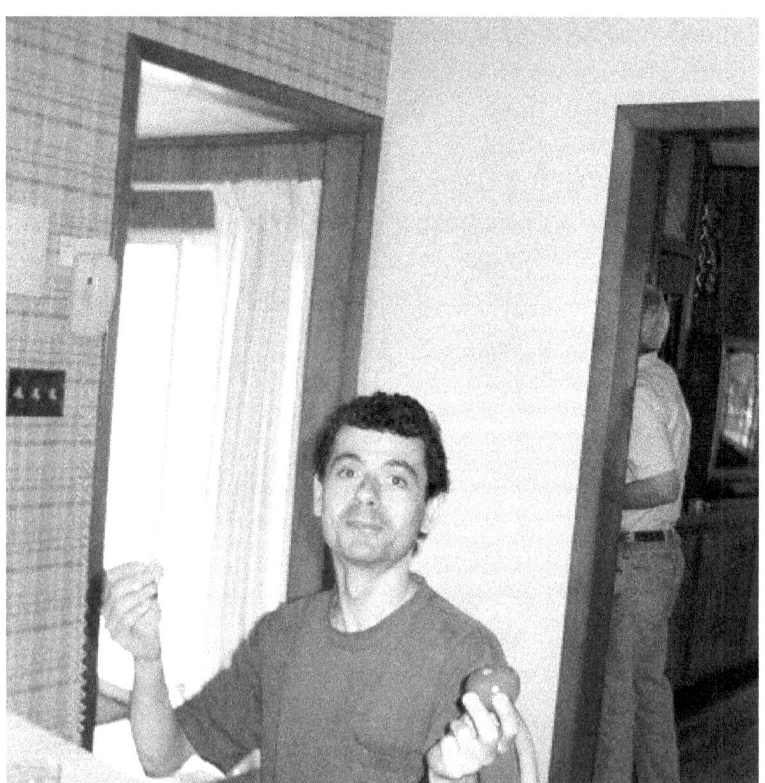

Roy at home.

"I need to do this," I told them. "I can't just bury my head in the sand anymore."

People needed to know the truth, and that was the end of it.

After Rhode Island, I went to Fall River and I spoke at Cedar Hall. Everybody was there. Anyone who wanted to come in, could come in. It went very well. People were coming up. They were like, "Wow, I didn't know it was that bad."

"Well, yeah," I said, "that bad."

Roy died in March, 2007

I look back, and in many ways I was probably a big disappointment to my father in that he was a cabinetmaker working around sharp tools and things of this type. I couldn't have been the son that he probably dreamed of having.

Francis Story

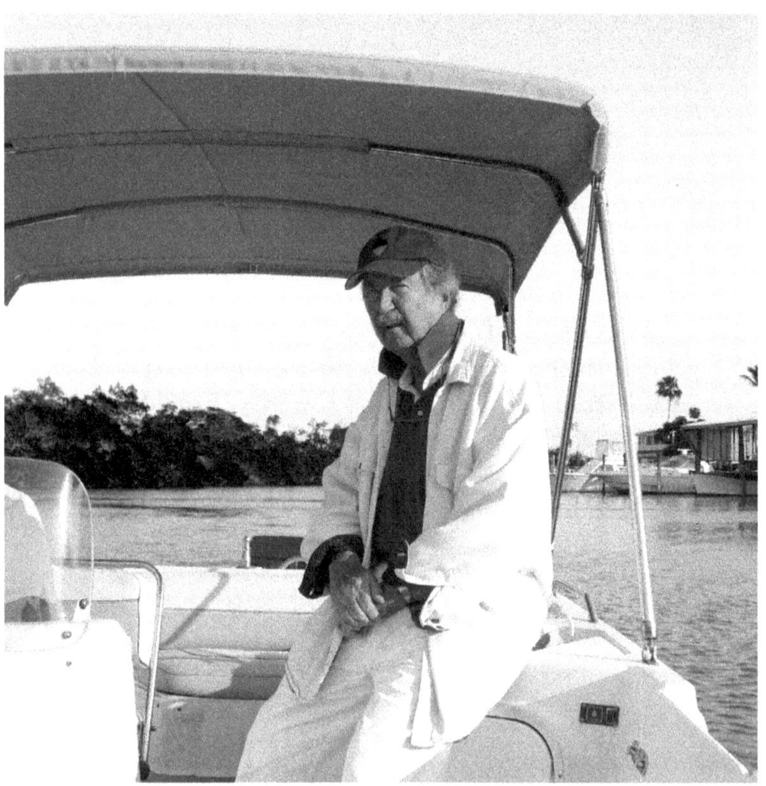

Francis has always been around and owned boats. Florida, February 2007.

FRANCIS STORY

Mr. Francis Story was born in 1928 in Beverly, Massachusetts. Sonny, as he is known, is married and has six children. He has grandsons affected with hemophilia. Sonny grew up during the Depression and has vivid memories of that time. He played in a band and ran an insurance company and is now retired. He has mild factor VIII deficiency.

I had a rare bleeding problem, hemophilia, that came down through my mother's side of the family. It was classified as the disease of royalty and my mother, bless her soul, loved to think in terms of luxurious lifestyle.

I have always felt that I can remember standing in my crib and hearing my mother hollering, "He's bleeding. He's bleeding. He's going to bleed to death." Fact or fiction, it's something that's always stayed in my mind.

We moved out to the country when I was about three, three and a half, four. It was a small, close-knit farming community and word got around.

"They have a son with a problem and he's bleeding," and so, in this close-knit community, I was known as 'the bleeder,' and you know, "bleeders don't live very long."

I was called Sonny, Sonny Story, and it was like, "If you play with Sonny Story, don't chase him because he might fall down and bruise his legs." At Halloween, it went around, "Don't let the air out of Sonny Story's father's tires because Sonny Story might get hurt and then his father won't be able to drive him to the hospital."

I ended up having a whole different lifestyle because I was the freak.

Back when I started school, in the first grade, you had to have a smallpox vaccination, but they didn't vaccinate me because of the fear that by scraping the arm they wouldn't be able to stop the bleeding. I've never had a smallpox vaccination.

In the sixth grade, I transferred from my small country school to the larger system, and when I got there, I was a total stranger. It was wonderful. Nobody knew me. I got rid of my nickname, Sonny, and became Fran or Frank, and I got rid of the tag, "hemophilia."

It was like a whole new world.

I still had to duck a few issues here and there. One was the fact that when my parents became involved, I tried to keep them in the background so they wouldn't tell anybody. I learned not to talk about my hemophilia. I felt that maybe it was a badge of dishonor. I didn't want to be looked upon as different, so I didn't talk about it.

The seventh grade opened up a whole new world for me.

At our little Christmas party at Sunday school – I must have been nine or ten – as a gift, the boys all got a jackknife and I, like one of the girls, got a coloring book. I couldn't have a knife because I might hurt myself. To this day, I always carry a pocketknife.

Amongst our grandchildren, you always hear, "Go see Grampy, he'll have a pocket knife."

I thought I was the best player in the class for Snatch the Eraser because nobody could catch me. Later on, I found out that they had all been told not to tag me too hard because I could get bruised. Everybody knew that I was a bleeder and they treated me special. I always tried to avoid the tag "bleeder."

I played hockey and I played fairly well, but my parents didn't know what hockey was. They thought it was something like figure skating, so I was able to get away with it until one day I really got whaled on the shin with a hockey puck. There was no camouflaging it after that. My leg swelled up like a balloon and then I went through a period when I wasn't able to walk.

Life was different in those days. It was a struggle to put food on the table. Men worked six days a week, and they didn't have Saturdays off. My father was out of the house to go to work before seven in the morning, he'd come home at noontime for lunch and then he'd come home shortly after five. He was a hard-working person.

I look back, and in many ways I was probably a big disappointment to my father in that he was a cabinetmaker, working around sharp tools and things of this type. I couldn't have been the son that he probably dreamed of having.

I had a cousin named Billie on my mother's side whom I never met, and they would say about me, "He's just like Billie." Then, lo and behold, at twenty-six Billie bled to death from a hit on the head. He was a debit man for John Hancock. Debit men went around the houses to collect weekly premiums and on his route, he encountered a drunk who hit him on the head with a bottle. So Billie went home and had severe headaches because he was bleeding internally. By the time they got him to the hospital, he was dead.

I tied into "bleeders don't live long."

"You can't do this and you can't do that because you'll bleed to death," and I pretty much locked into that.

"Well, if I could live to be twenty-six, you know, I'd be really lucky."

So I'm on the plus side of life. Anything beyond twenty-six, I was on the plus side. Right now, I'm fifty years on the plus side.

My brother had hemophilia. During the Depression, my father was having difficulty feeding the whole family, so the people who were keeping my brother said, "Gee, why don't we keep him a little bit longer?" It was agreed that that was the best way to handle the whole situation.

It was kind of a strange upbringing. My brother and I were separated at a young age, and for many years I was told I was the only one who had hemophilia. I was told that my brother did not have it, but then it showed up in him when he was about fourteen.

Nose bleeds would occur in the middle of the night. I'd call to my mother and she would come in and she'd panic. I could understand why she would. When we ran out of handkerchiefs, she'd tear up sheets and pillowcases.

My father would always say, "Margaret, you'd better take care of it, because I can't stand the sight of blood".

My teeth had to be extracted, and they did it by taking a little piece out at a time. I'd develop terrific clots in my mouth: a clot would grow and grow and grow, and it would keep growing to the point where I would have a whole

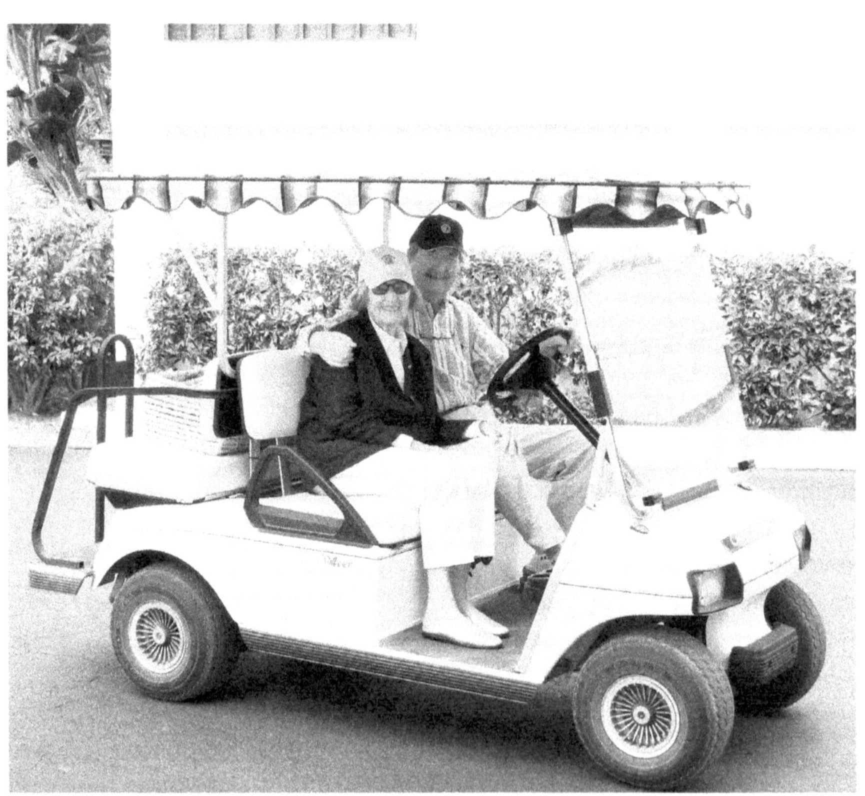

Francis and his wife, Mae, in Boca Grande, Florida in 2007.

mouth full of blood clot. Then we'd call the dentist and I'd go back and he'd have to scrape it all down and start over from scratch on the clot process.

This happened day in and day out for almost a week, until, finally, fraction of an inch by fraction of an inch, I was able to get the cavity where the tooth came from patched up and the clot would hold.

They treated the bruises and the joints by way of bandages, like Ace bandages. They would bandage me up or put a splint on my leg. If they didn't, it would keep swelling and swelling and swelling, then I'd be bedridden. I had to keep my leg elevated, sometimes for a week, two weeks.

The other thing they did was to give me a heavy diet of liver. Whenever I had a nose bleed, my mother cooked up liver like crazy and it would be almost raw. She'd put it in the frying pan and flip it over, flip it again and then I'd have it. You'd think I would hate it, but I enjoy liver, to this day even, cooked that same way.

They'd feed me a lot of cod liver oil and liver extract, which is the worst tasting medicine in the world. Terrible, terrible, but it was important to get my iron level up.

I didn't want to be labeled 4-F, but I was told that I would never be able to go into the Navy because I had hemophilia. Later on, I thought, "Well, if I don't say anything, they're not going to know. They're not going to know until I'm in."

From my standpoint, I was saying, "I'm one of the guys. I'm the same as everybody else who's going off to war. It's the patriotic thing to do."

There was a period when everybody wanted to play the trombone like Tommy Dorsey. I was always interested in the drums, but I said, "Well, gee, maybe I might like to play the piano, too, or a wind instrument." I was told to rule out playing the trumpet or the trombone because I had hemophilia, and blowing into the instrument could start a bleed internally.

I mention this as one example of the crazy things I was told.

"Everybody in the company has had approval on their thousand dollars' worth of life insurance except you, and it's because you have hemophilia."

Right away I said, "Oh, geez, does this mean I'm going to lose my job?"

It turned out I didn't lose my job. I went on to become the head of the company.

It's amazing, absolutely amazing, how closely people associate hemophilia with AIDS. In a minute, you can see it in people's eyes. Mae might say "You know, Fran has hemophilia," and you can almost see people recoil. You just know, and it's not my imagination. People do.

I had a bad accident this winter down in Florida and people were saying, "Geez, I've always heard of hemophilia, but I've never seen anybody with it."

Then I heard somebody in the hospital say, "You ought to go down to see the man in that room, he's the oldest living person with hemophilia in New England."

You don't want to be labeled in life, you know, and wear a Scarlet Letter.

I think if I had dwelled on the disease, there would have been a lot of avenues in life that wouldn't have been open to me. Things wouldn't have been possible for me. As it is, life's been wonderful. I've had six marvelous children. I have five daughters and a son who does not have hemophilia. He is a DEA agent, off on drug raids and jumping out of planes. He lives quite the different type of life than I do.

My mother is a caring person. It's not as though she had us live the way we did because she just didn't want to deal with it. It was because she cared enough.

Michael Donovan

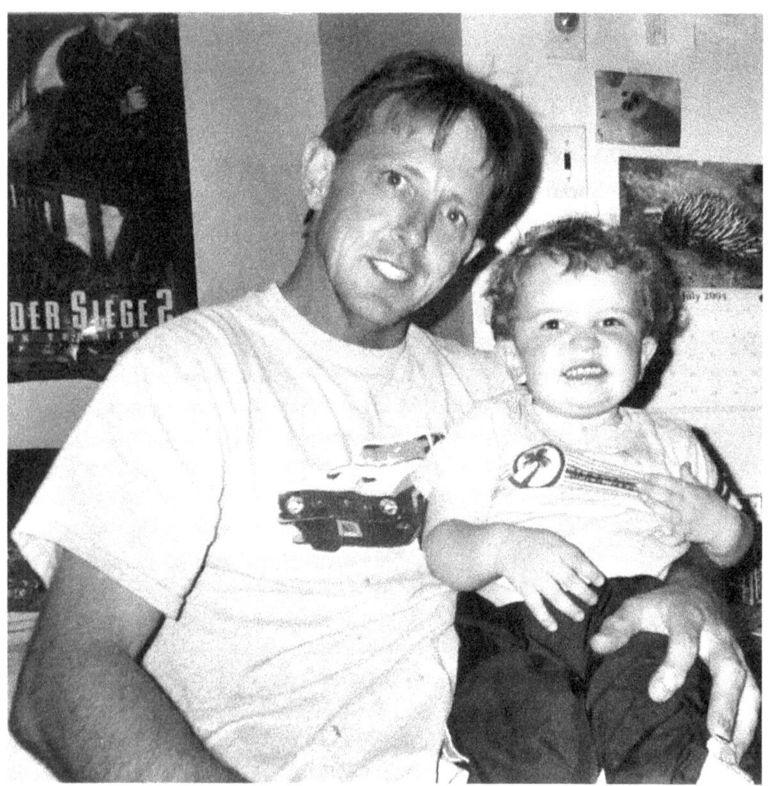

Michael with a young friend, Jack.

MICHAEL DONOVAN

Michael Donovan was born in Boston, Massachusetts in 1962. After his father left the family, Mr. Donovan's mother moved to Houlton, Maine and, later, to Whitman, Massachusetts, where Mr. Donovan went to school.

He has a degree in electronics and has worked for many years in auto repair at a dealership. One of his two brothers passed away from HIV.

Mr. Donovan is not married, travels at every opportunity and enjoys competing in poker tournaments. He has moderate factor VIII deficiency and hepatitis C.

My father left the family when I was four or five years old, and my mother worked two jobs after he left in order to take care of us. When I was a kid, she drove a school bus and then she did other things, too. She had some other small jobs.

As for my father, he was gone.

They found out that my brother, Tommy, had hemophilia. Once they knew he had it, they checked and all three of us had it.

The doctor at Children's Hospital in Boston who first diagnosed my brother told our mother not to baby us. He told her not to limit our lives, so to speak. Obviously, we weren't going to play professional football or anything, but she raised us not to let hemophilia limit us.

My mother actually helped me enjoy my life instead of living afraid. I met some people at a charity softball game this summer. They were all so scared about their kids and what was going to happen. Once they knew I was forty and had hemophilia, they really wanted to ask me a lot of questions, but I'm not the person to answer those questions because I didn't do what your average person with hemophilia does. My mom made sure that we didn't not do this or not do that. Was there a risk? Maybe. But did we limit our lives? No.

My mother gave me a gray area, so to speak. It wasn't yes or no. It was kind of "Well, give it a whirl and see what happens."

My mother is a caring person. It's not as though she had us live the way we did because she didn't want to deal with things. It was because she cared enough.

When I was young, in the '60s and '70s, treatment was pretty harsh. It's nothing like it is now. You were given a large quantity of a frozen plasma-type substance; that's the best way to explain it. It was put into you cold. It made you cold, and if the nurse or whoever was giving it to you administered it too quickly, it made you really ill. I remember that from when I was, like, four. It's something you never forget.

Some nurses were a little bit more compassionate about a four-year-old getting an injection, and other nurses were just in a hurry and wanted to get on with their jobs. That's just the way it was.

I can probably understand what it would be like for the parents because I saw what it did to my mom.

It's a good thing our mother was strong enough to live with us. I think about what it was like for her when I came in with blood pouring off me or bruises this big or broken bones. I mean, I've broken a lot of bones. I've broken bones and not had an injection. I've had bruises that went from here to here and didn't go for an injection. I just never wanted them.

I've always tried to avoid the injections whenever possible. I've only had them if I absolutely had to. That is probably why I'm still sitting here in front of you.

Should I have taken the injections? Should I have gone to the hospital every time I hurt myself? Would I have the pain I have now if I had done that? But then again, would I have gone rock climbing? Would I have played hockey? Would I have roller bladed? Would I have done everything I've done if I had lived a different way? Probably not. So, yes, it was the right thing for the doctor to tell my mom.

His advice gave me a life. I'm not saying that people with hemophilia don't have a life, but if you walk on eggshells, your life is going to be limited.

I have no fluid left in my joints. I've been going to a specialist and it isn't going to get any better. It's just going to get worse. If I'd known that twenty years ago, I don't know whether I would have taken injections, because my brother,

Tommy, died in '84, '85 of HIV from an injection. Back then, when you got HIV direct from a blood product, you died quickly. It wasn't as though they had a lot of medications to slow it down.

We weren't raised to run to the hospital. I'd have to be really hurt to go. It was called life and you dealt with it and you went home with it. The support network was the family and we helped each other when we needed it.

That's one reason why, when I do go to them, doctors think that I'm not quite on the up and up, so to speak. They don't know what to think because I don't run to them for every nick and scratch, every ache and pain. When I go, I'm hurting. You know what I mean?

I have pain in my elbows, my shoulders, any joint you can mention. I'm arthritic. I have severe bone spurs in both my ankles, which has limited my mobility. Eventually, it's going to become zero mobility, but once that happens, the pain in my ankles should diminish. I just had arthroscopic surgery on my knee. You're supposed to have a layer of liquid between your joints, and I basically have zero in my ankles at this point. I've had cortisone in my shoulders several times already. I wake up in pain and sometimes I can't adjust to it.

I said something to one of my doctors and he said, "Well, you just don't like doctors, do you?" It's not that I don't like doctors, but there's always a gray area when you have hemophilia and you go to a doctor who's not a hematologist.

How many forty-year-old hemophiliacs are there? Not many, so nobody really knows what it's like to be a forty-year-old person with hemophilia.

My doctor is kind of worried about me taking pain medication now because I'm only forty, and it's going to get worse. When I was going to my other doctor and trying to explain the pain I was in, he didn't understand hemophilia.

They kicked me to the curb for years.

I've recently become involved with the Hemophilia Association at Brigham & Women's, and Dr. Bell and the other people there actually know what a forty-year-old hemophiliac feels like. At least there is somebody who knows.

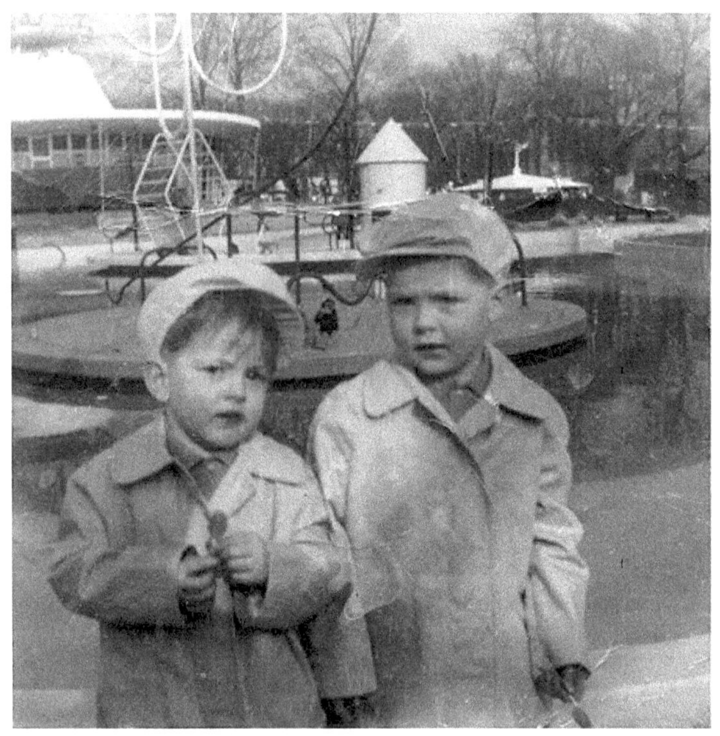

Michael (left) and his brother at the Franklin Park Zoo, near Boston, about 1969.

I applied for the military. There's a medical form you have to fill out and as soon as they saw hemophilia on it, they said, "No." They obviously didn't want me.

It's not like everybody in the military has to be on the front line. I'm a mechanic. Shouldn't it be my option, if I want to take the risk myself? But if you're a hemophiliac, you're not getting into the military. Back then it was pretty cut and dried.

I got a degree in electronics and I'm in the electronics end of automotive repair. I'm happy with my professional life except, again, I've got to reflect back on the pain issues I have now. I'm on my feet ten hours a day.

I don't know how many years of work I've got left in me, but hemophilia did not stop me from doing what I wanted to do. I probably should have gone into something that didn't involve using my body as hard as I use it, but I didn't. I'm happy; I'm good at what I do, so I don't second-guess that decision.

I have $30,000 worth of tools, so wherever I go, if I take them with me, I won't be unemployed. I'm staying home now to take care of my mom. I don't have a big social life. I don't date a lot, obviously, because that would be the worse thing at this point in my life.

I can live with the physical pain, but, you know, getting older alone is going to be real tough.

I'm forty-two now and when I look ahead, I'm figuring fifty. To be blunt, it isn't anything nice. I have a good life. I have people I care about and they care about me. I heard that I lose ten to fifteen years right off the rip just having hemophilia. Then I got the bad blood from whomever and that isn't going to help me down the road either.

I guess maybe that's another blessing, that I'm not waiting 'til I'm sixty years old to enjoy life.

I'd rather have a good moment in time instead of a piece of jewelry. I'd rather be taking my nephew A.J. to the Caribbean and just walking downtown. To me, that is something I'll remember forever. I mean, a watch — I can get another one. I do all right at my job, but that's not the way I live.

I travel all the time. I do everything now because who knows? I play in

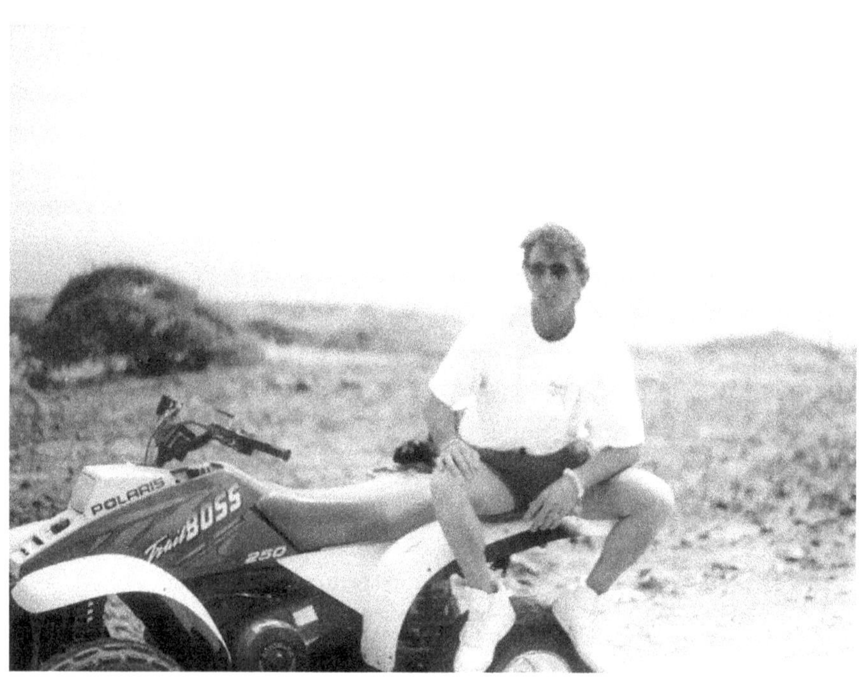

Michael on vacation with his family in Aruba.

poker tournaments all the time. I actually play online and win a lot. I finished 50th out of about three hundred last time, and those are people who play religiously, so I was happy.

I just spent a lot of money to fix the heater in the house, and I'm going to take my mom to Vegas next month for three days. You know, I've got to get mom out.

In some ways, it's been a gamble all along. There have been some pretty scary things in life, you know, but we were never raised to be afraid. If you're raised to be strong, that's a big help in life, even if it does end a little bit sooner than everybody else's.

No matter what I do or how I live my life, eventually it's going to catch up with me.

I'm not a very religious person, but I guess I'm spiritual in a way. I'd like to think that there's more to it than some of the things that are dumped on people on a daily basis. I'd love to think there's something better in store for people who aren't as fortunate in life as others.

I really do believe that things happen for a reason. Maybe my not being here 'til I'm sixty is going to affect somebody else in a positive way. Or maybe my disease, something that's happened to me, is going to do something for somebody else.

I — and the people in my family — have a lot to offer somebody. I'm a very fair and giving person. But if you decide not to be in my life, then that's your prerogative. I'm not going to chase you. I wish you were in my life, but if you don't want to be there, then I can't make you be there.

I try not to dwell on what might have been. I look at what tomorrow brings me. Sometimes, I can't help thinking about things, but most of the time it's momentary and I get right back on with my day.

Those guys from the pharmaceutical companies sit sipping margaritas on a yacht in the Caribbean, and I haven't dated in five years because of what happened.

The pharmaceutical companies claimed no responsibility for any of it. My mom received some money because my brother Tommy died, but she didn't get rich, believe me. It wasn't a huge amount, and because it was due to my brother's death, she didn't really want it. But, like I said, everything happens for a reason.

Maybe Tommy died so my mom could have a comfortable life. I guess if you want to, you can look at things that way.

Things could be worse.

I mean, every day you see people who have got it a lot worse than I do. What? I'm going to live a little less and deal with a little pain? You know, it's all right so long as I do the right thing every day and I can put my head on the pillow at night and know I did the right thing.

If somebody else wants to bitch about something minor, then God bless them because they should probably find something to divert their attention, just so they're not miserable their whole life. You know what I mean?

Why would I blame my mom because I have hemophilia? She gave me life. So what if she had known that she was going to give me hemophilia and not had me, then I wouldn't have had any life at all?

FINDING THE CAUSE*

In the 20th century doctors looked for the cause of excessive bleeding. Until then, they had believed that the blood vessels of people with hemophilia were simply more fragile.

1930s

Doctors previously thought defective platelets were the likely cause of bleeding disorders. But in 1937, doctors at Harvard University found they could correct the clotting problem by adding platelet-free plasma. They called the substance "anti-hemophilic globulin."

1940s

In 1944 Dr. Pavlosky from Buenos Aires, Argentina, did a lab test which showed that blood from a person with hemophilia could correct the clotting problem in a second person with hemophilia and vice-versa. He had stumbled upon two patients, each with a deficiency in different proteins - factor VIII and factor IX. This led to the eventual recognition of hemophilia A and hemophilia B as two distinct diseases. By the end of the decade people with hemophilia had a life expectancy of less than 30 years. Treatment was limited to icing joints where internal bleeding occurred and painful transfusions of whole blood.

1950s & 1960s

In the 1950s and early 1960s, hemophilia and other bleeding problems were still being treated with whole blood or fresh plasma. Unfortunately, there were not enough factor VIII or IX proteins in these treatments to stop serious internal bleeding. Many people with severe hemophilia, and some people with mild or moderate forms, died in childhood or early adulthood. The most common causes of death were bleeding in vital organs, especially the brain, and excessive bleeding after minor surgery or trauma. Those who survived were often crippled by the long-term effects of repeated hemorrhages into the joints. The pressure of massive bleeding into joints and muscles made hemophilia one of the more painful diseases. By the mid-1960s the clotting factors were identified and named. An article in *Nature* in 1964 described the clotting process in detail. The interaction of the different factors in blood clotting was termed the "coagulation cascade." In 1965, Dr. Judith Graham Pool published a paper on cryoprecipitate. In a major breakthrough, Dr. Pool discovered that the precipitate left from thawing plasma was rich in factor VIII. She found that because cryoprecipitate contained a substantial amount of factor, it could be infused to control serious bleeding. Blood banks were able to produce and store the component, making emergency surgery and elective procedures for hemophilia patients more practicable. This advancement also ended the need for high-volume whole plasma transfusions for people with hemophilia.

1970s

By the 1970s, freeze-dried powdered concentrates containing factor VIII and IX became available. Factor concentrates revolutionized hemophilia care because they could be stored at home, making treatment easily accessible. People with hemophilia could now "self-infuse" factor products, drastically reducing the number of requisite hospital visits. Activities such as work and travel were now carried out with much greater ease, the benefits being increased convenience and independence.

1980s

Although hepatitis C was already present in the blood supply, by the early 1980s a new blood-borne disease would emerge. By the mid 1980s, it had become clear that HIV/AIDS could be transmitted through the use of blood and blood products, such as those used to treat hemophilia. Approximately half the people with hemophilia in the U.S. would eventually become HIV-infected, and thousands would die. The overwhelming impact of HIV on the hemophilia community would reverberate well into the next decade.

*Courtesy of the National Hemophilia Foundation, 2007

I really think that the families dealing with hemophilia adjusted in the same way families of children with other serious illnesses, such as leukemia, adjust. What was very important for these families was the trust they had in the people taking care of them.

Dr. Herbert Strauss

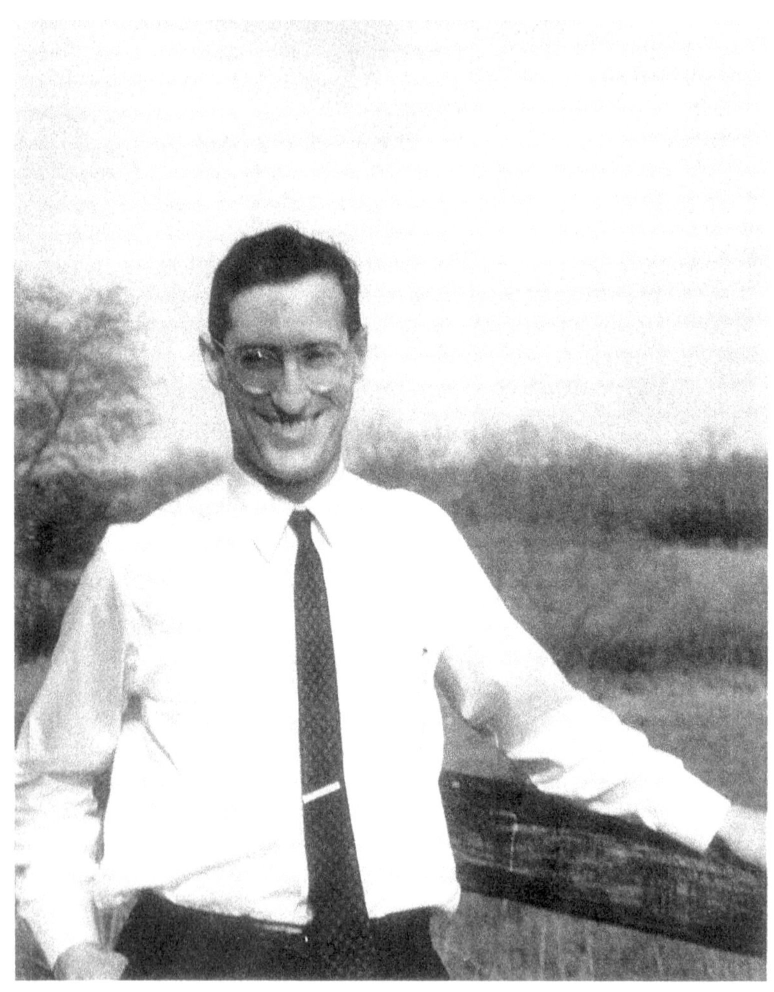

Dr. Herbert Strauss

DR. HERBERT STRAUSS

Dr. Herbert Strauss was born in Frankfurt, Germany, and moved to Palestine when he was six. He attended medical school in Zurich, Switzerland. Among his influential professors was the internist, Wilhelm Loffler; the pediatrician, Guido Fanconi; and the psychiatrist, Manfred Bleuler. In 1954, Dr. Strauss immigrated to the United States. After a rotating internship at Michael Reese Hospital in Chicago, he completed two years of pediatric residency at Queens General Hospital in New York City.

Dr. Strauss was drafted into the military and served for two years as a medical officer at the U.S. Naval Hospital in Beaufort, South Carolina. There followed a one-year fellowship in pediatric hematology with Dr. Doris Howell, a former fellow of Dr. Louis K. Diamond's at Duke University in Durham, North Carolina. From 1960 to 1969, Dr. Strauss worked in Dr. Diamond's coagulation lab at Children's Hospital in Boston, chiefly occupied with issues surrounding hemophilia. In 1969, Dr. Strauss moved to Albany Medical College in New York. Since 2001 he has been living in retirement in Saratoga Springs, New York. He and his wife have two daughters who live and work in the Boston area.

Dr. Diamond offered me a job in 1960 in the clotting lab at Boston's Children's Hospital; this was a very unique position at that time. In most places, if you were in the lab, you were in the lab. You provided tests; you got requests for this and that test; you gave the results; and the clinician took care of it. With Dr. Diamond, it was different. The laboratory was totally funded by research grants. When there was a problem with bleeding, they called us: we went there, took the history, found out what was needed and devised our own clotting tests. That meant that every problem had to be solved, just like detective work.

Dr. Campbell McMillan, my mentor, was already in the lab when I arrived. We worked together very well. Both Campbell McMillan and I were interested in improving the care, not just doing what was standard care at the time. We were searching for improvements and finding new facts about hemophilia.

We were paid a pittance, but I was not married so it didn't matter that much to me at that time. We were available to the patients at all times by phone, whenever there was a problem, in the way that old-time physicians were always available.

The standard care then was to give fresh frozen plasma for factor VIII deficiency and bank plasma for factor IX deficiency. For episodes of hemorrhage, we infused fresh-frozen plasma. We had great assistance and help from the Orthopedic Department under William T. Green, who was very dedicated to the care of hemophilia. Joints distended with blood were always drained. Joint aspirations were done under completely sterile conditions in the Operating Room, then the joint was immobilized with casts, followed by gentle mobilization with help from Physical Therapy. This elaborate procedure, though difficult, was very successful.

I distinctly remember one eleven-year-old severe hemophiliac who was repeatedly admitted to the hospital for joint or muscle hemorrhages. Going through his charts, I figured out that this boy had cumulatively spent a whole year out of his life in the hospital. He was not disabled; he had no muscle contractures or joint deformities. If he had not received this painstaking treatment, he surely would have become disabled.

The Dental Department was also helping us. Dental care was very important for the hemophilic patients, and often required local anesthesia. This required needling, meaning that the patients had to be protected against hemorrhage. I remember one severely affected teenager with inhibitors. He could not receive local anesthesia because we could not protect him with factor VIII. General anesthesia was out of the question because that would have required intubation, which could have induced life-threatening hemorrhage into his neck. It so happened that the Dental Department knew of a dentist at Tufts who was expert in hypnosis. He sat at the head of table with the patient, talking softly and reassuring him. The dentist did some deep drilling that must have been painful, but this patient lay there without making a sound. I was deeply impressed that hypnosis really worked.

In the '50s, the group at the University of North Carolina in Chapel Hill (UNC), which included Drs. Langdell, Brinkhous and Graham, had invented a test they called the Partial Thromboplastin Time (PTT). I learned of this test while spending a year at Duke University in 1959 and 1960. When I came to Boston, I introduced the PTT test to Children's Hospital. This PTT test is now used universally.

The PTT can miss mild cases of hemophilia. The Thromboplastin Generation Test, TGT, is much more sensitive and specific for deficiencies of factors VIII and IX, but it is a more complicated test and requires training and great dexterity to perform accurately. With the TGT, one was able to diagnose even the mildest hemophiliacs, whereas without this test some milder hemophiliacs escaped detection.

Most textbooks of internal medicine or pediatrics state that about 30 percent of hemophiliacs have no family history for hemophilia. The fact that over ninety percent of the sporadic cases are severely affected and that almost all the milder cases have a positive family history, is not mentioned. I published a paper about this in 1967. It was entitled "The Perpetuation of Hemophilia by Mutation," and was published in the *New England Journal of Medicine*. No one had come across this fact previously.

Back in the early 1960s, several European pediatricians and hematologists thought that eating peanuts was helpful in protecting hemophiliacs from bleeding. A drug called epsilon aminocaproic acid (EACA) was also thought to have similar beneficial effects. Dr. Sherwin Kevy and I did a controlled study with eight severe hemophilia patients; our results proved that giving patients EACA made no difference in the incidence of hemorrhage. We published our findings in the *New England Journal of Medicine*. After that publication there was no more talk about eating peanuts or giving EACA as a way to reduce the incidence of spontaneous hemorrhages in severe hemophiliacs.

Following the discovery of cryoprecipitate by Dr. Judith Poole, Dr. Sherwin Kevy prepared cryoprecipitate in our blood bank at Children's Hospital. We used fresh normal plasma, froze it, then thawed it slowly and got this gunky material, rich in factor VIII. That led to its use for prophylaxis. I think we were among the first people to use cryoprecipitate for prophylaxis. Our program of infusing cryoprecipitate every 48 hours was totally effective in preventing spontaneous hemorrhages. I assumed this protocol as self-evident and regretfully did not publish our findings.

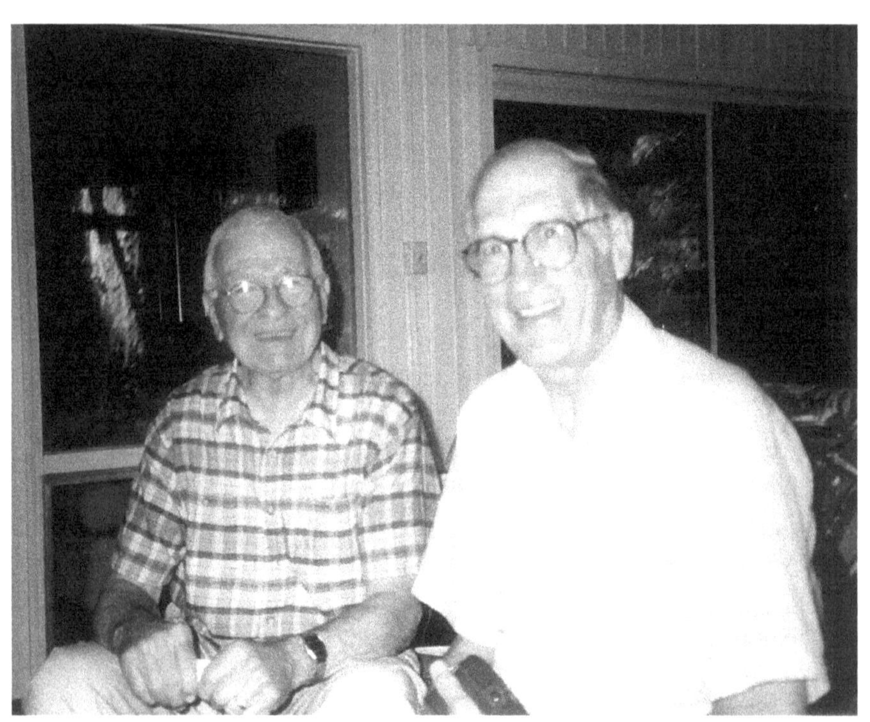

Dr. Campbell McMillan and Dr. Herbert Strauss at a reunion in Chapel Hill, North Carolina in 2002.

In regard to the discovery of cryoprecipitate, I'm always reminded of the discovery of penicillin. Many clinicians observed that contaminating fungi often inhibited bacterial colonies on their petri dishes, but it was Fleming in England who used this observation to discover penicillin. I can say the same thing, in a much more modest fashion, about cryoprecipitate. When thawing tubes of frozen plasma, I often noticed gunky stuff floating in the plasma. I considered it a nuisance and shook the tube to dissolve the material. That was cryoprecipitate.

I should have been curious enough to say "Well, let's see what's in there. Let's centrifuge it down, separate it and test it for factor VIII and see how much factor VIII is in it."

I studied the natural history of the factor VIII inhibitor over several years. I recorded the days on which patients received factor VIII, and any day they received factor VIII was counted as an exposure day. I found out that all the patients who developed an inhibitor did so before reaching 95 cumulative days of exposure. Any patient who escaped developing an inhibitor by the time he reached this critical exposure subsequently failed to develop an inhibitor. This was of huge significance to patients who were on regular prophylaxis.

The treatment of patients with inhibitor was very difficult. I set up a factor VIII inhibitor assay that proved important for the treatment of these patients. Knowing the current inhibitor levels of our patients and their individual responses to more exposure to factor VIII allowed a logical approach to handling dangerous hemorrhages.

Treating hemophilia patients was challenging and also very gratifying. When a hemophilia patient arrived at the Surgical Outpatient Clinic bleeding massively, we needed to get blood in a hurry. I ran to the second floor blood bank! In order to give blood you have to do a cross-match. An adequate cross-match takes half an hour. Sherwin Kevy would do an emergency cross-match, which took only two minutes. Perhaps this was not a hundred percent reliable, but that's the best we could do. By the time I got back to the clinic carrying a bag of blood, I'd call the blood bank: "Is it okay?" and then we could start using it. And I mean, I would run. I wouldn't wait for the elevator. I would run up to the lab and then run down to the clinic. There was this close fusion in those days of lab and patient care and research. Everything was intertwined. The research was related to the care, the care was related to the lab, and so on. It was a unique situation, and it was interesting.

There was a lot of implicit pressure to do studies, publish or perish, to justify my position, so to speak. There was always this pressure to do more than just take care of patients. I think I have done some valuable things, things that I am happy about — my two articles that were published in the *New England Journal of Medicine*, the article on mutations in hemophilia in 1967 and the article on the factor VIII inhibitor in 1969, were my most valuable contributions.

To quote Goethe, "Blut ist ein ganz besonderer saft" (Blood is a very peculiar fluid). Blood has many functions, including the delivery of oxygen and the transport of many substances. It is also our central heating and cooling system. When the limb is too hot, the circulation opens up and there is more blood flowing for cooling. When the limb is very cold, there is constriction of blood vessels to reduce the blood flow and save heat. A child in need of an IV may have collapsed veins and one is stymied inserting a needle. So what do you do? You put the hand in a basin filled with water as hot as can be reasonably tolerated for a few minutes. Blood vessels open up. The blood flow into the arm is increased dramatically. Then you take the hand out and put a tourniquet on the arm. Now the veins are engorged and you can easily slip a needle into the vein. I have always encouraged house officers to use this procedure.

I really think that the families dealing with hemophilia adjusted in the same way families of children with other serious illnesses, such as leukemia, adjust. What was very important for these families was the trust they had in the people taking care of them. They trusted those caregivers to be consistent and available. Having people really interested in them and really taking care of them — that's important. You often don't have that anymore.

It's nice to hear that my name still comes up from the patients I treated. That's good to hear, because it's nice to be appreciated for trying to do one's best.

It is noticeable to me when I am free of pain.

Andrew Flagg

ANDREW FLAGG

Mr. Flagg was born in Massachusetts in 1959. His father was a plant manager at a plastics firm and his mother was a bookkeeper. He has two older sisters. His grandfather died from complications of hemophilia when Andrew was eight years old.

Mr. Flagg took his Bachelor's degree in biology in Boston and his Master's in biology in Ohio. Married with two step-children, he works as a medical writer.

Mr. Flagg has severe factor VIII deficiency, HIV and hepatitis C.

I've always felt fortunate to have been born near Boston and that I was able to take advantage of those resources, even though it meant my poor parents dragging me into the hospital at ungodly hours. They're not the best trips, those that you do in the hours of darkness.

Apart from specialists, back in the '60s there was not really great awareness about hemophilia. Even though I knew my options were better than if I had grown up in many other places, it was not uncommon to go to the Emergency Room in Boston and be asked, "How long have you been a hemophiliac?"

"How long has it been a problem for you?"

That really does tell you that they don't know about the disease.

There is still an awful lot of management in my life as opposed to just doing. Apart from the life-threatening issues, the almost complete lack of spontaneity is the biggest drag. You always have to be aware of the consequences of not paying attention for a minute or two, and that weighs pretty heavily.

The first thing you notice with a bleed is the loss of range of motion. Just a few days ago, without knowing how, I hurt one or two fingers, enough that I noticed I couldn't move them quite as well as I wanted to. I must have bent them back shoveling. Those little things happen all the time. I had to reschedule this interview, for example, because on that day my ankle wasn't good.

That is probably the second biggest impact of my hemophilia, that on any given day there's something that ranges from a little bit annoying to disabling, a condition that won't allow me to walk, for example. That extreme is rare, but there is always something that's limiting, and it's unpredictable.

Pain has been a huge problem because it's isolating. If you're in pain, you're just not open to a lot of things. Pain is the biggest problem, aside from not being able to physically do things or being confined to bed. There are very few times when I'm not in some kind of pain, and that's been true since I can remember.

It is noticeable to me when I am free of pain.

It's definitely easier now, from a management point of view, than I thought it might be. The advances in treatment have been huge. They don't show up with these enormous syringes any more. In earlier days, the nurse would come in with a 50 ml syringe, and I remember saying to my mom, "I'm feeling better now."

Pain even isolates you from your family because you don't really feel like making the effort to be sociable. All you really want is to be more comfortable.

Being in more or less constant pain affects your behavior and your approach to life.

My initial reaction to being asked to do something – and this is purely a reaction – is "No," because I'm starting from pain. I'm already in pain and I don't want to add more.

The pain and the limitations have forced me to slow down and I think that has some benefits in the way I look at life. I am more aware of what's going on in the moment. To this day, I always look for things I can do while I'm in a recliner or some other ridiculously elevated position, because that makes a big difference.

You find yourself in cycles where it's impossible to recover entirely. One joint hurts, so you tend to compensate with the another joint, then that gets sore and leads to a bleed. It's a constant push and pull.

As we speak, I have a couple of joints that hurt and won't work that well for me, so my balance today is different from my balance yesterday. You always have that.

It's hard to get back to being fully recovered.

I had one particular experience in relation to pain in my knee. I can see it as we speak. I was sitting quietly in a chair, thinking about the pain but not thinking that I wanted it to go away. Only one other time in my life have I ever felt so calm. I was thinking about it, but I wasn't fighting it.

There was one other time when my wife and I and the two kids were going to my parents' house on an Easter Sunday. I was getting out of the car and I haven't felt a sense of calm like that before or since, a sense that everything was okay. It has stuck with me all these years.

It kind of tugs at me, that maybe that feeling is still around somewhere.

I always had one or two really good friends at school who would come over to my house. People would help me keep up with the assignments. In high school, I had to leave class a little early in order to get to the next one, so I was always very popular when I needed someone to carry my books.

I didn't find much prejudice among my classmates, but sometimes they would ask me how it felt to have hemophilia.

"So, if I punched you right now," one kid asked me, "would you bleed?"

I said yes, and he punched me.

Fortunately, he punched me in the arm and muscle bleeds are not a big deal. Over the next couple of days, I showed him the effects of what he had done.

I think if people have a preconceived notion, it is that if I cut myself I'm going to bleed to death and it will show.

I remember a *Time* magazine article that came out when I was in high school saying that the average age at which hemophiliacs died was twenty-one, or some ridiculously low number. I mentioned it to my mother and she said something like, "Oh, are you feeling sorry for yourself?"

Looking back, that was the right answer.

Insurance coverage is the biggest determinant of what I do, I would have to say. I can't do without it: I either have to find it or get lucky. The health insurance part is pivotal. Both my parents had health insurance and I was covered as long as I was under twenty-five and a full-time student. I intended to go to graduate school, but I wouldn't have minded taking a break right after college. Because of health insurance, that was not an option.

I earned my Master's, and I was still twenty-fourish when I came back to Massachusetts. I actually enrolled in a junior college to bridge the time until I could get my own coverage. That was very weird. I literally started at junior college the day I came back from getting my Master's, and that was all because of health insurance. Junior college wasn't wasted, though, because I took a course in technical writing and now I'm a medical writer, so it didn't hurt.

The insurance companies would never tell you directly that you were covered, not over the phone and certainly not in writing. As it turns out, I was always covered, but you didn't hear that in advance. You could look through all their information, but you could never get someone to say, "Yes, we'll cover you for home infusion of factor VIII." It always feels as though the situation could change at any time.

When I apply for jobs, I don't always bring up the fact that I have hemophilia unless I think it's really relevant. I did interview with someone for a lab position and I must have mentioned hemophilia because he called me back and said, "You know, we use a lot of glass plates in our lab work and sometimes we have to score and break them."

I assured him that wasn't a problem.

In my head I was thinking, "I didn't go to all-plastic universities you know."

I am HIV positive and there's no way to estimate the amount of concern that's caused me, even though personally I have not had much difficulty as a result of the diagnosis. I haven't had complications, but there aren't many days, if any, where it doesn't cross my mind.

The big impact of HIV, aside from the concern about getting sick, was the feeling that I needed to go underground again. There was an article in the *New York Times* magazine by a hemophiliac who had essentially the same reaction. He was starting to feel more comfortable about his hemophilia as a man and a person, then, suddenly, because of the HIV, it wasn't something he wanted to tell anybody. He didn't know when or how he should bring it up.

There's always the feeling, "Well, I seem to be doing okay, but I'm one blood test away from finding out that I'm not doing okay."

My wife and I have worked it out, but I'd be curious if you could ever actually be honest with yourself or another person as to how much of a concern the health issue actually is. My wife has never really expressed that, but I can't imagine that it isn't a concern for her, in the same way that, in the back of my mind, it's always a concern for me.

The fact that, day-to-day, I don't know whether I will be able to do something has been difficult on my marriage. It is very limiting, but I think as we get older it's less of a problem. My wife and I met twenty years ago, and when we got together she already had kids, so she had plenty of things to worry about other than whether I could go skiing or not. I would like to be able to walk more, though, because that's key.

There's something about us just walking together.

I actually feel that if I can stay in the same shape I'm in now, I'll eventually be pretty much on a line with my peers. I look around at guys my age and I think, "I'm probably doing okay."

Then there is this irony. Here's the factor that can give us life and it might, at the same time, take it away. The new irony in the making for me is that if you have hepatitis C and have a liver transplant, you may no longer be a hemophiliac because the transplanted liver might produce factor VIII. That's happened at least once.

I can't even begin to think about that.

I am hopeful, from a purely selfish point of view, that gene therapy or other types of therapy will emerge that can, if not cure, at least provide managment of this disease. I hope, again from a selfish point of view, that medical advances might lead to a cure because I would really enjoy not having to think about it for a little while.

It really is with you every day.

My dad died five years ago from the complications of lung cancer. I think of this all the time. He had decided he wasn't going to have any more procedures to help them figure out what was going on, but then they said, "If we do this one procedure, maybe we can figure it out."

"Wouldn't that be joyous?" he said, even though he was tired of going through it.

That was the last procedure he ever had, but even at that point, after all he had been through, he was still hopeful that this procedure would tell him something.

The outcome is not a fairy tale, but my dad's attitude coupled with "We'll find a way," is something I think about all the time.

My mother was the same way – "We'll figure it out" – and that has translated into my life. I think it has to do with how they grew up. My dad grew up with nothing, not even a great family life. When I think back on what he didn't have and what he was able to do, that impresses me. My mother had a pretty good childhood. Their experiences informed the way they were.

I think my parents did a great job of starting me off with a good chunk of self-esteem. I'd much rather deal with a sore knee and feel that I'm probably okay otherwise. And I can feel joy.

"Well, it's a sore knee, I can't go skiing." That's not such a big deal.

I've had my right knee replaced and my right ankle fused and I could really use matching surgeries on the left side at this point. It's made a world of difference. The pain in my right knee, in particular, was constant, and now my left knee's getting to the same point. You've seen it before; you know it can be fixed, but until it gets to the point where it's bleeding or there's some weird opportunity to take three months off work, I'll probably let it go another year or so.

I don't think I've really ever had depression. I've been lucky to always be around good people, people I want to be with. Maybe I can't always do what I'd like, but I'm happy to be with that person.

What actually prevents me from feeling more calm or happy at any given moment? It's probably looking ahead at something I'm not looking forward to.

I'm actually a little bit proud of what I've done.

Despite all the physical limitations and dealing with things like HIV and the unknown hepatitis C, I do think I'm relatively okay. I should be proud of that, rather than feeling afraid to have people find out about my limitations. I think I'm doing okay with everything that's gone on in my life, whether people know about it or not.

I do know that people have no idea how difficult it is.

Hemophilia is part of you and there's no differentiation. It's not added on after the fact, you don't have a sense of self or identity and then something's layered on. Hemophilia is about as much a part of me as my eyes and my breath, so I don't know any different.

It wasn't like "This is hemophilia."

"This is me."

Avida - "To go with life"

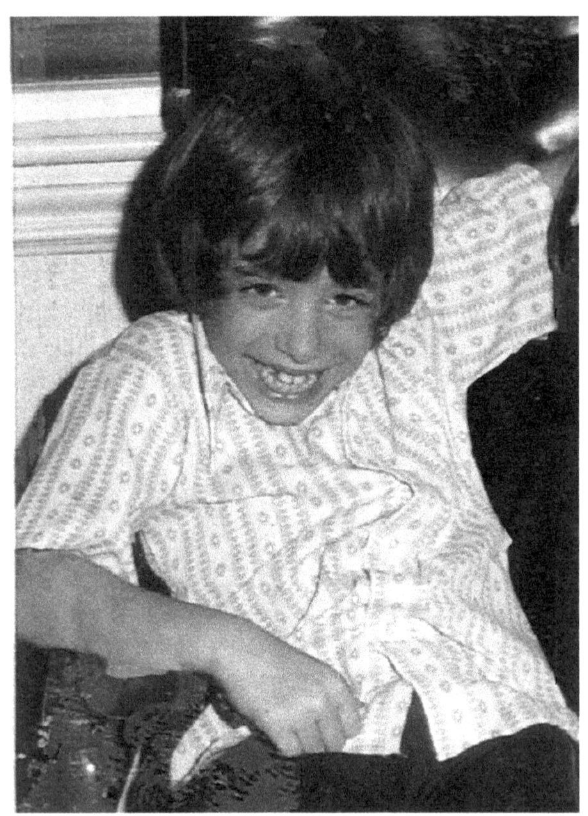

Living in order to live.

AVIDA

Avida was born in Massachusetts in 1964. At the age of nine, he moved to Michigan. Avida has an advanced degree in psychology and is currently working to grow a nonprofit community arts and wellness center in Massachusetts.

He has severe hemophilia, HIV, hepatitis C, is healthy and has happiness (5-H Club) in his life.

My father died in '78, when I was fourteen. I was old enough to remember him well, but we didn't get into discussions about hemophilia. That said, I'm forty now and I really haven't talked too much with my mother about it either.

I was not one to be very open. I have the capacity and with certain people I am open, but in my family I don't have any memories of what you would call conversations that went right to the core issues of fear and sadness. It can be nothing more than "I'm sad, hold me." I was encouraged to be a strong boy, to be a good boy.

My parents were not over-protective at all, far from smothering and far from being negligent. I think they tried to let me have as much of a so-called normal life as possible. I didn't play football, but I was never really interested in it. I played baseball. I ran around. There are pictures of me as a kid in kneepads.

I didn't feel restricted at all. I rode my bike, fell off it, got treated when I did. Cuts and bruises and scrapes aren't going to do anything. In terms of the effect on the family, I think the stress was great, particularly the pressure on my mother. She's the one who always had to take me into the Emergency Room, long before home infusion.

You were at the mercy of the system and there wasn't much mercy in the system. I don't know that I've ever trusted medicine, once I realized what it was. People creep into the system, and they're not bad or incompetent, they just don't have enough sensitivity. They're not the right people for the task.

I'm not saying that anyone was purposely scary or purposely mean, but it was as though someone yanked me out of my home, put me in a strange space with strange sounds and started doing things to me. You don't know what's happening and there's not necessarily a calming period first, so there's distance. You're in pain and someone's helping you, but you're still in pain. You don't understand. Your mother's there. Your mother—your protector, your caregiver, your intimate, your love, your creator—and yet she's brought you into this horrific place and you only feel better a good time later.

Relief is far from instantaneous. It was hard to make the connection.

I don't think I really understood at first that the treatment was making me better. What happened to me seemed like a brutal procedure. I can't even imagine what that experience was like for me as an infant. I know that I was strapped down. Sometimes my arms were held down, just to get the needle in, a functional procedure, but not necessarily done in the most humane way. My sense is that unless there were exceptional parents and exceptional medical caregivers, most people with hemophilia back then, and maybe still today, were traumatized as infants.

You can't escape the pain. It's just everywhere. Even though the pain is in the joint, it is just in you and you can't work with it, at least I wasn't able to at times. But there seemed to be a point—I don't know how old I was—less than ten, when I came to an understanding. I reached a threshold where the pain became routine. It feels like the first time someone gets mad at you or you fall out of love. There's an understanding that comes with the experience.

Hemophilia is part of you and there's no differentiation. It's not added on after the fact, you don't have a sense of self or identity and then something's layered on. Hemophilia is about as much a part of me as my eyes and my breath, so I don't know any different.

It wasn't "This is hemophilia."

"This is me."

This discussion is probably the most I've ever talked about hemophilia in my life. It's never been much of a discussion with friends, because to me it's a matter of fact. I don't know anything else. It's just present.

I don't remember being ostracized by others, but sometimes you'd almost ostracize yourself. The disease changes your persona. It makes you more withdrawn, quieter and you do other, less active, things.

⁂

Having hemophilia has limited me in many ways. You can say there are always things that limit you, but there are basic things I'd love to do that maybe I can't. Fortunately, I developed a fairly positive attitude somewhere along the line, in fact, I think I've always had that. I'm not compulsively happy, far from it. At times I'm sad, serious, very realistic, but I've always been able to see the beauty and engage it.

⁂

Nothing really terrible has happened. I deal with pain every so often. All right, it goes away. It's not that bad. My father died. I grieved and got over it, although I miss him and I miss all the opportunities to engage him in my life. It's not that these things don't impact me, but I'm alive and I'm vital and I'm feeling and sensing and being and growing and changing constantly.

When that process stops, that's when it becomes hopeless.

⁂

I remember reading something about HIV when I was in college. For some reason I thought I had HIV, but I didn't really know what it was. I had a fever or a rash. I went to the student clinic and told the doctor and he said, "No, you have none of the signs. Everything's fine." I didn't think about it again, forever.

⁂

At some point – I don't remember what year – it became a reality that people with hemophilia were being diagnosed with HIV. One of the main things that that growing awareness impacted was my exploration of sexuality and love. Love, really and mainly.

I responded with fear.

"I can't get into a relationship. How am I going to meet someone? How are they going to deal with this?"

I didn't know. I still don't know.

I denied that part of myself out of fear. This is at the beginning of it all, and there was the stigma and the idiocy, the lack of acceptance and the sense of being ostracized, that surfaces when anything scary like HIV comes up.

I started going to school in 1987, and the people at the clinic there were surprised I hadn't been tested. Every time I went to the clinic, they'd say "You still haven't been tested?"

I'm like, "Why do I have to get tested? What's it going to tell me?"

yes

health

happiness

hemophilia

hiv

hepatitis c

"Then you start therapy." You know, the whole spiel.

Finally, just to get them off my back, I said, "Fine, I'll get tested. I don't care." In my mind, it made no difference. It wasn't going to change a thing, but now I was going to know. I had to live with that fact, even though I knew anyway, kind of.

So I was tested. This is '91, and there were probably only a few people who hadn't been tested at that point. I was positive. At the clinic, they were long-faced and I was like, "All right." In some sense, knowing beforehand, then actually hearing the diagnosis and dealing with it, was kind of scary.

Right after that, I met a woman, and we grew a love relationship together. Obviously I told her from the beginning, and I was amazed by what she said. She was concerned about my health, but it didn't really impact our relationship. I mean it did and it didn't. She didn't retreat.

That was a huge awakening for me. It's not that I don't value myself or see who I am, but there are only so many things anyone wants to take on with another person. We were both young. I can see not wanting to deal with things like alcoholism or a chronic disease, never mind something that might well be terminal.

HIV has a stigma, so of course it impacted her. She was tested every year. They encouraged testing just to be certain, even though there was no way anything was going to happen.

Every woman I've been with since — three other women, two and the one I'm with now — they've been amazing. I still don't get it. Every time I have to tell someone that I'm HIV positive, I'm sure they'll run away or retreat. It still blows me away when they don't. You see so much fear and running away in day-to-day life that when you're confronted with the opposite, it's a little mind-boggling, and inspiring, too. So these women have all had huge hearts and they followed their natural emotions. They did not retreat from their love or from me.

Things are as safe as they've ever been, that's true, but a bullet's still a bullet. Any disease can creep in at any time.

There was a period when I was just finishing up in graduate school, when I thought I'd be lucky to live ten years. That was the thought I was living with: at times, it was devastatingly sad, but most of the time it was just a reality. I don't think that awareness brought me down, but it changed things.

I was going to retrain in clinical psychology, which was awesome, but it was a three-year program and I might only have ten. Why was I going to the trouble if I could only practice seven years? It didn't make sense to me, so I totally changed my life course, still operating under the belief that I was going to die.

That thinking had a huge impact. It changed my life.

I've never had faith in an organized religion to guide me, lead me, sustain me, support me, but I don't feel at a loss. My mother feels it's a loss, but I've had faith in my way. My faith is more just in living, in what's present in our being.

I think the darkest moments really occurred at the beginning of the acknowledgement of HIV, when I changed what I was going to do. My father died at forty-two and before HIV, I had a goal, kind of half joking, but real, to live longer than my father. It's two years away now, but I didn't think I was going to make it to that point until four years ago. Now I don't know, just like anyone doesn't know, but I don't think I'm going to die soon. I'm not making decisions based on that.

In those darkest moments, it's like grieving. It's a sadness, a reality you work with and grow through. At some point, it became less troubling to me that I was going to die in ten years. I had to go on with my living now, because I had ten years – maybe. That was good. Some people don't have ten years.

The lawsuit. Some people probably should be in jail, if you talk about crimes against humanity. That was a crime against humanity and financially it was a joke. The drug companies got off easy, but people accepted it. We accepted it. The law firm accepted it. That's the way the system works.

The settlement has been extremely important and it's given me the freedom to do some things. I just wanted to add that, because it's a very big part of the picture for a lot of people.

I think the reality of hemophilia, at least for my generation and before, is that the worst is yet to come as we grow older. No one prepared me for that. No one even mentioned what would come later and that seems to me to reflect some degree of ineptitude. So much faith is placed in drugs that no one ever said "Be happy you're alive." There's a sense that everything is being taken care of, but the pain that I have now in terms of arthritis is way beyond anything I had with joint bleeds.

The disease is as active in me in some ways now as it's ever been, but it's all secondary. It's only recently that it sunk in that what I have is degenerative. I'm not having joint bleeds much at all, but the damage done earlier is here with me now, loud and clear.

Either you go with the flow, or it drives you nutty. You have to accept it, and if you accept it, then it's just a way of life. If you don't accept it, then it's going to cause a lot more problems. That's the way I ended up looking at things, and that's how I always made it through.

It was, "I'll take today as it is, and whatever tomorrow brings, I'll deal with it."

Cliff Deschenes

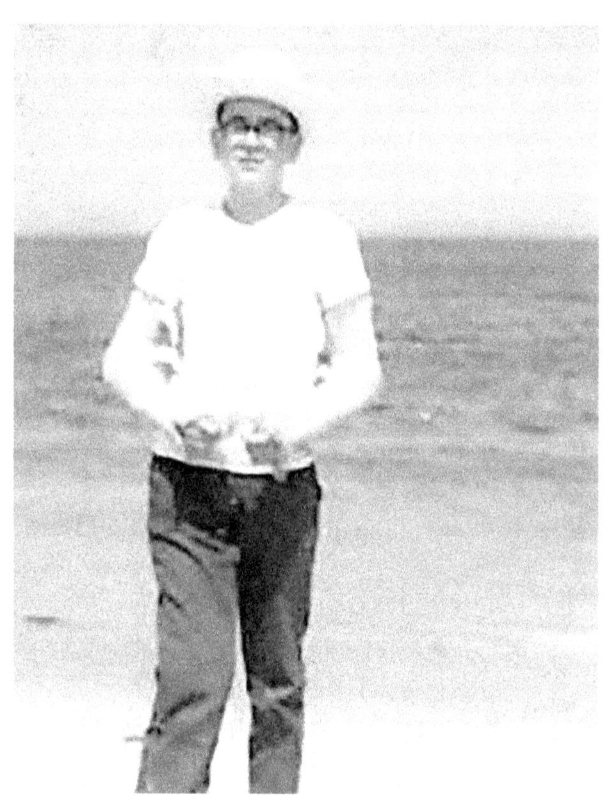

Cliff at the beach, age 12, with two arms and one leg in casts.

CLIFF DESCHENES

Mr. Cliff Deschenes was born in 1954 in Lawrence, Massachusetts. He works in electronics at Wang Laboratories and is married with two children. One nephew has hemophilia. He has learned to take one day at a time so as not to get too frustrated. Cliff has severe factor VIII deficiency, HIV and hepatitis C.

When I was in grade school, I was in the hospital quite often, at least every other month. I'd be there anywhere from a week to two weeks for a bleed.

They didn't have the treatment they have today. If you had a bleed, you had to be admitted to the hospital because they had to use plasma and there was so much volume that it took hours and hours to drip through.

My dad always used to take me in if I had a bleed. He'd stay with me until I was settled, then he'd go back and do what he had to do. He came every night. Every night. He'd go to work all day and then, after he got out of work, he would drive all the way back into Boston, stay with me until eight o'clock, then drive all the way home.

If my parents resented it a little bit, they never showed it.

My parents were protective. Basically it was, "Don't do this. Don't ride bikes. Don't play sports. Don't run." There were a lot of restrictions, and if you abided by them, you probably didn't get a bleed as often.

I have pictures at home where I have a double leg cast and an arm cast or two arm casts and a leg cast.

A lot of the time the doctors couldn't get an IV started because, in those days, I was fat. In the second grade, I weighed a hundred and twenty pounds. I was as high as I was wide. Dr. Strauss would say, "You don't need all that weight."

If the doctors couldn't find the vein, they'd try once, maybe they'd try a second time, then my dad would say, "That's it, no more. You don't get a third shot."

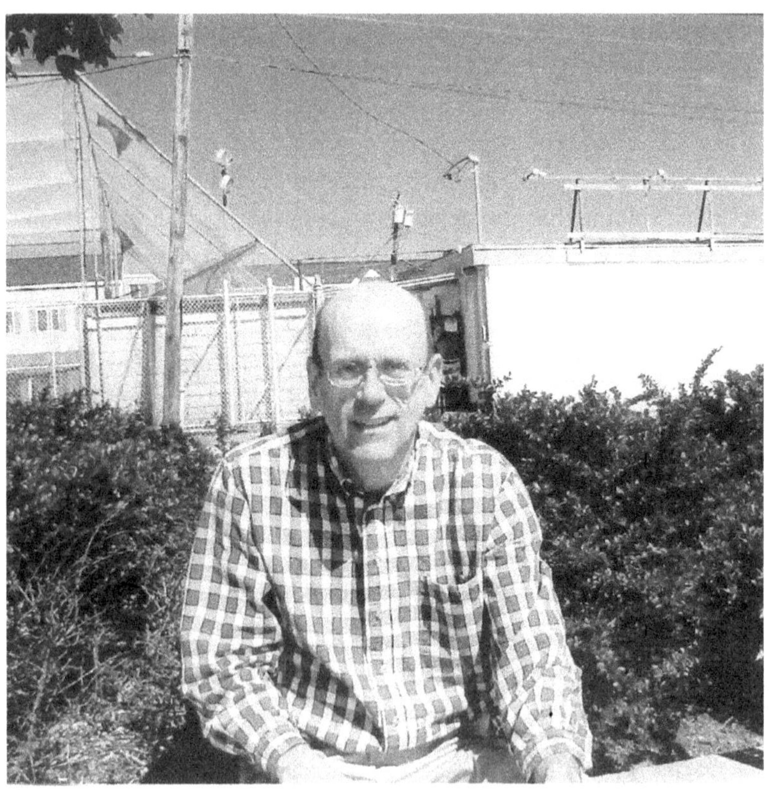

Cliff at the beach, age 50.

Nobody wants to go to the hospital. "I'll hold off. I'll hold off, just be quiet, don't tell", but after awhile they'd notice. Either you couldn't use an arm or you weren't walking too well and it was like, "What's bothering you?"

Oops.

Often during recess I would just stay in the classroom and the main corridors of the hallway. You weren't supposed to run in the hallways, but I was racing kids up and down on my crutches. It was something I had to do, and I just did it.

There were always other kids in the hospital room. They may not have had hemophilia, but they had their problems. Seeing other kids with different problems, I used to say, "I'm not too bad because he's worse off than I am."

Either you go with the flow, or it drives you nutty. You have to accept it, and if you accept it, then it's just a way of life. If you don't accept it, then it's going to cause a lot more problems. That's the way I ended up looking at things, and that's how I always made it through.

It was "I'll take today as it is, and whatever tomorrow brings, I'll deal with it."

I was always included. It wasn't as though I was excluded because I had hemophilia. If my family did something, we all went. If they went to the beach, I went to the beach, and many of the times I was at the beach, I had casts on.

About the time I went to high school, they started offering prophylactic care. That meant being treated every other day but, at the time, you couldn't do it at home. Every other night, for two or three years, my dad would get out of work, pick me up and we would drive all the way into Boston Children's Hospital.

In the Emergency Room, they'd give me all the paperwork, then I'd go up to the Blood Bank. The people there knew me on a first-name basis, and it was like, "Okay, it's over there in that refrigerator."

I'd take my cryo back to the Emergency Room, then I'd have to wait around for a doctor.

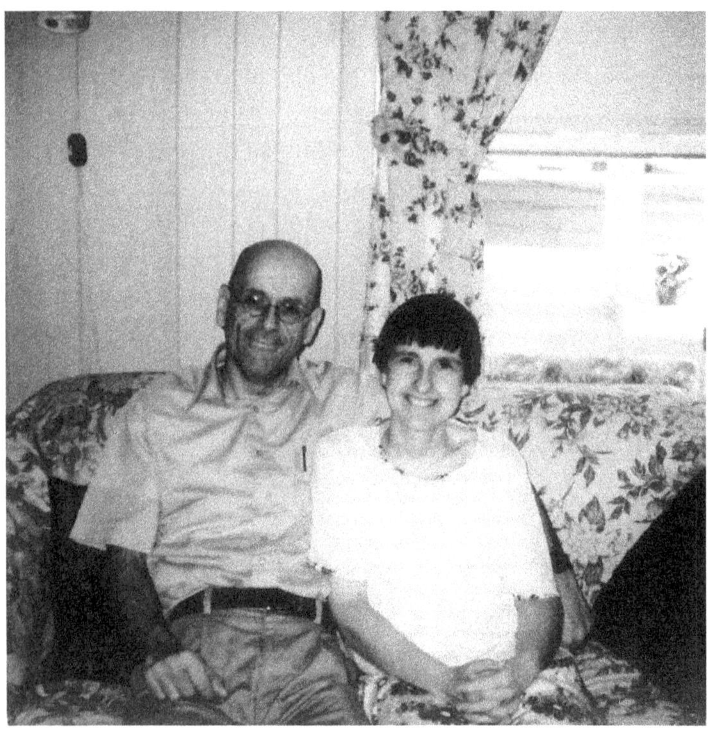

Cliff at age 51 and his wife, Jayne, at home.

The doctor asked me if I wanted to learn how to administer it myself. I said, "Sure."

She gave me her arm and said, "Here, put the needle right there."

So I put it in on the first shot and she said, "Okay, next time, come and see me, I'll let you do it yourself." After that, I started doing it myself every other night.

I was brought up Catholic and one of the things a Catholic believes in is God. I believed that if I couldn't handle it, He wouldn't have given me what I have.

You've got to be able to have something in your mind that helps you get through. It may not be a God, it might be something else, but it's a spiritual thing. You've got to reach a different level to handle this.

A lot of pain is in the mind. It's physical, but you can control a lot of it with your mind. You can't eliminate it, but you can make it less severe.

Back then, when I was thirty years old, if you were getting blood products, the odds were you would be infected with HIV. My wife was afraid she would get it and it was rough for a while. Oh, I cursed it a little bit: "Why? Why did I get this?" But then, I went back to, "Okay, I can handle it."

Doctors kept saying, "You should go on treatment," and I would say, "Why?"

"Well, because your T-cell count is 500," and I would say, "It was 500 three years ago, so give me a reason why I should be treated."

"Well, a normal person's supposed to be around 1500 for the T-cell count."

I answered, "I'm at 500. I've had 500 forever."

They kept asking, and my T-cell count at the time was going down. It went down into the 200's. I finally told them, "I'll go on treatment when my T-cell is below 200. Then we'll discuss treatment."

The way I looked at it, there's always a chance of getting something if you're taking drugs. If you want to treat what you've got, there's a chance you might get something else. Damned if you do, damned if you don't. You've got to go down the road and say, "Well, this is what I have to do now and I hope it works."

Most people who have something wrong with them from the beginning, end up accepting it. They don't let it really bother them because it's part of their lifestyle.

⁂

The company hired me, then called me up an hour later and said, "Oh, we can't hire you." I couldn't really do anything about it, but I knew what the reason was. They'd read my medical history.

⁂

When you're told you can't do something, you say, "Watch me. I'll do it."

I still have that same drive. If somebody challenges me to do something, I'll try to meet the challenge.

One day at a time. Some days it's not a day at a time, it's an hour at a time. You go an hour at a time and you say, "Okay, I made it through that far, now go a little further."

You pray that you can handle what is being dished out. You pray for the intelligence, the common sense, the ability to handle what isn't working right, or even sometimes maybe just to be thankful for what is working right.

Jeryl Drummey

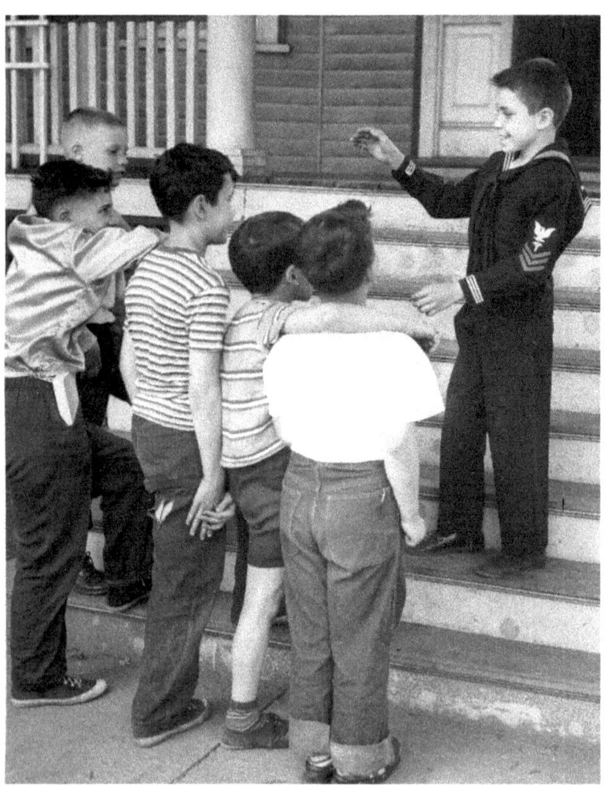

Boston Globe photo taken in 1950 as part of a Children's Hospital fund-raising campaign. Jerry is on the right in the photo.

JERYL DRUMMEY

Mr. Jeryl Drummey was born in 1941 in Brighton, Massachusetts. Married with one daughter, he worked for ten years in a book store and then for twenty-five years for a distributor of women's clothing. Jeryl feels strongly that health providers must treat the person and not just the disease. He has moderate factor VIII deficiency.

When I was four, going to the hospital wasn't always a very pleasant experience because back then most of the doctors knew very little about hemophilia. Unfortunately, many of the doctors thought they were going to discover all about it, and, frankly, they didn't know what they were doing. They would aspirate the swelling. They'd take a large-gauge needle, stab it into the joint and squeeze the blood out of it in order to get the swelling down.

Extremely painful. They'd give you a little novocaine, which wouldn't do anything. And I mean, to start with, the joint was bad, then to take a needle and just stab it in like that — and when I say stab it, they'd raise the needle over their heads. They would take the fluid out, then the next day, of course, the joint would just fill up again.

Twenty times or better I was kept over in the hospital. It's hard to say. It seemed like a long time, but it was probably a week or something like that. As a child, it seemed like a very long time.

It was not Children's Hospital as it is today. It had old bungalows out back in the days when they actually had some property with grass on it. They didn't even have elevators, so when they took me into the hospital, they had to carry me upstairs.

You could feel the plasma when they shoved it in. You could feel it go right up you. When it was still cold you could feel it right through your gums.

I was having a lot of pain. They gave me some codeine to fight the pain, but then there was one doctor who tried passing some sugar pills off on me.

"Take these," he said, "these will be better. These are very powerful. These will control the pain completely."

Jerry Thanks Donors

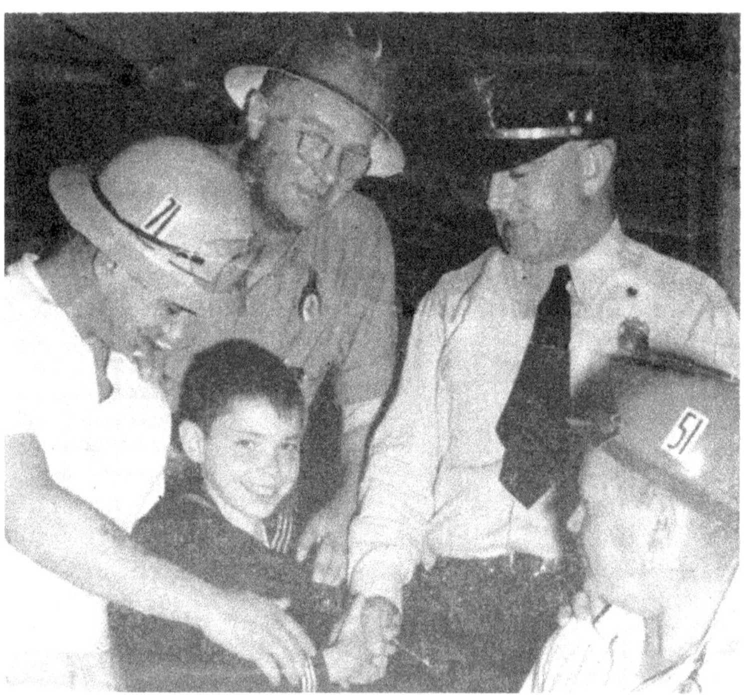

JERYL DRUMMEY, hemophilia victim who is the son of James V. Drummey, sandblaster, Paint Shop, chats with Albert Dutra, Walter Gordon, Assist. Police Chief Donovan, and James Bell. Jerry came here to thank all blood donors for their help.

He was going to prove something: "Well, I can control the pain just by giving him sugar pills and he'll think the pain has gone away."

When we saw Dr. Diamond later on in the afternoon, he took a look at those pills and he was furious.

Physical therapy was a problem back then. I was having a lot of trouble with my left arm. The physical therapists didn't understand hemophilia and what caused problems, so they kept forcing exercise and usually, by night, I'd have bleeding in it again. When I began physical therapy, I could only straighten my arm so far; by the time I got through with physical therapy, I could straighten my arm a whole lot less.

I kept running into people who had different ideas; they didn't really understand what they were doing. That created a lot of extremely bad experiences for me until finally, one time, they wanted to aspirate again and I said, "No, that's it."

"I'm out of here," I said, and I left the hospital. I left the whole system for years.

Maybe God is watching over me. Maybe it wasn't all my decision. Maybe He helped me make it. For some reason, I made the right decision then; I went the way that I felt was the way to go. It wasn't anything about HIV; it was just that I was not being treated right. That's why I left and I just picked the right time to do it. Maybe it was luck. Whatever it was, I'm glad I made the decision then.

So many people my age just aren't here now because they stayed in the system.

There were a lot of very good doctors who did a lot of very good things for me, but unfortunately I remember the bad ones a lot better.

One time I had an infection in my foot. This was way back when you could actually go swimming in the Charles River – believe it or not, there was such a time – but even then it was pretty polluted. I cut my foot and it got infected. I had to go to the hospital. The infection was bad; they admitted me.

They woke me up in the middle of the night and all of a sudden they were holding me down and cutting into my foot without any kind of anesthetic. That's why I have a lot of bad feelings about hospitals and doctors.

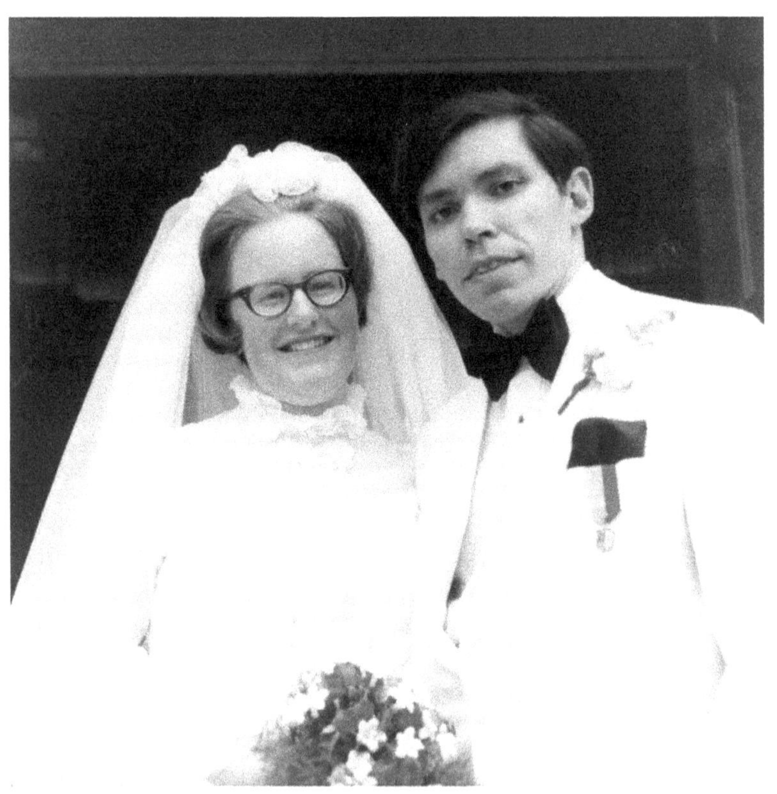

Jerry and his wife Kathy on their wedding day in July, 1970.

I got to the point where I had to make my own decisions on most things and figure out what was going to be the best thing for me to do, not what was best for someone else. I learned that my doctor is working for me; I'm not working for him. His job is to do what I need. I've got to use his intelligence, but I have to use it in the context of my needs and what I really require, not as a patient, but as a person.

I think the only thing the doctors and social workers, the nurses and the family must remember, first of all, is they are dealing with a person and not a hemophiliac. You can't just treat hemophilia; you've got to treat the person. That has to be primary.

You can't just say, "We're going to treat hemophilia and that's the only thing that counts." It's not. If the treatment becomes more important than the quality of life for the individual, then the treatment isn't worth anything.

I never went to school; I had all my schooling at home. The school system was afraid to take me because I was a hemophiliac. They were afraid something would happen to me and they might be held responsible. I went through all twelve grades at home.

To me, it was just a normal way of life. I never thought, "Well, gee, it could have been different." That was the way it was. If you don't accept who you are and try to do what you can with what you are, you're not going anyplace.

Having hemophilia made me think a lot more about how to do things. I had to look at the risk and figure whether the risk was worth it and what I wanted to do. You have to weigh everything and then you go ahead and do what you want to do, if you can.

I was cautious, but I did a lot of things. To me, the quality of life, in terms of what you can do, is a very important thing. I mean, if life is all about what you can't do, then life isn't too great. I wanted to fly a plane, so once I was eighteen, I took flying lessons, and I did get a license.

People said, "Oh, no, you can't. Too dangerous. Too dangerous. Don't do it." But I did and I learned to fly and that was a fun part of my life.

The person's quality of life is the important thing.

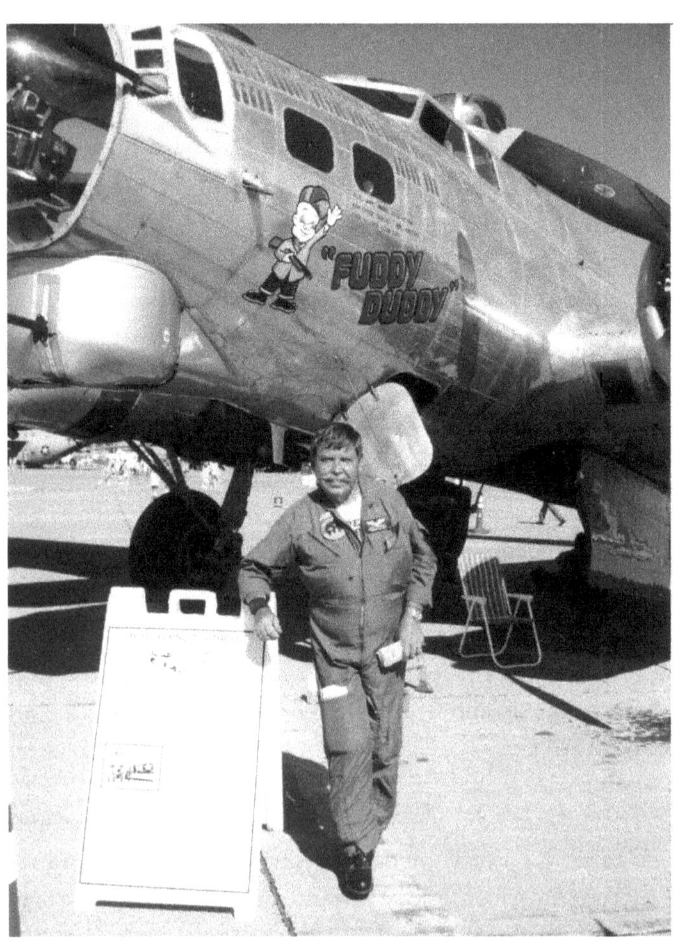

Jerry conducting tours of a B-17 Flying Fortress at the Niagara Falls Air Show, June 1977.

I was at a support meeting, and met the parents of a boy who had hemophilia.

"Do you think it would be a wise thing," they asked the doctor, "when our son eats if he uses a spoon because he might hurt himself with a fork?"

I remember thinking that the poor kid was going to grow up eating with a spoon the rest of his life.

Find out what the child wants to do in life, what he wants to achieve. Don't be too quick to say, "You can't do that."

There's always a problem when you really can't do something, like you're having trouble with your legs, you can't walk and you can't go someplace. That's the downside. Now I will often do as much as I can. When I'm feeling fine, I will sometimes push very hard just to enjoy every minute, because that's the upside of life. You just enjoy all the good moments you have and that way you don't have that many bad moments.

You're not going to face life unless you go out and do it.

We're all handicapped in one way or another.

If you want to compete in a prize fight, you'd be handicapped against a professional.

I guess where you are weaker in some areas, you are probably stronger in other areas.

Few people really understand hemophilia, how one time you can be in very bad shape and a couple of weeks later, you can be just fine and have no signs.

Most people, unless they have hemophilia, don't really know what it's like. It's not until you have it that you know what it does, what it can do and what it can't do, what's a myth and what's not a myth.

Pain is an old and disagreeable friend.

Enemies don't hang around that much, but the pain stays. I've had it for some sixty years in one form or another. Even though I don't like it, I have to sort of consider pain my friend because it sticks with me.

The fortunate thing about pain is that you can forget a lot of it. You remember pleasure very well, but pain — fortunately, the mind blocks a lot of it out.

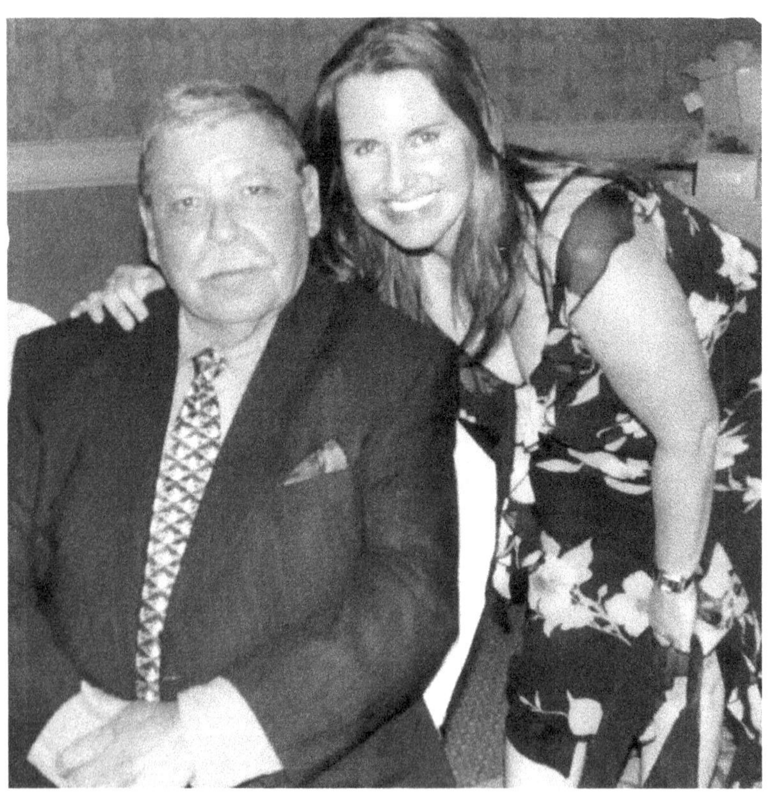

A current picture of Jerry with his daughter, Anne.

You can remember, "Boy, I had a hard time. I couldn't sleep for three days because there was so much pain." But you don't really remember exactly how the pain felt.

You pray that you can handle what you are being dished out. You pray for the intelligence, the common sense, the ability to handle what isn't working right. Sometimes you pray that you will be thankful for what is working right.

"But for the grace of God, it could be me." And at times it was me, so I welcomed the chance to help other people with a problem, to do something to help them and make their life a little bit better.

Religion is a solace and a comfort when things are really bad and everything seems to be going wrong. It's a comfort, something you can lean on a little bit.

First my wife had to marry me, then she had to marry hemophilia.

That was me and this is me. First you have to like me, then you have to like or dislike any of my problems.

They told me I don't have to worry about having an operation. Earlier in life, an operation was a no-no — you didn't do surgery on people with hemophilia. I started finding out more and more about factor and when I had the hips done, it worked out very well. Then I found out that physical therapy had improved, that there are therapists who know what they're doing. I called my physical therapist Attila because she put me through torture, but it was for a purpose. She did a great job. My hips are really good.

Hurt is a part of life. You're going to get hurt sooner or later.

1990s TO PRESENT*

Treatment for hemophilia and other bleeding disorders advanced in the 1990s. The safety and efficacy of factor concentrates improved. Factor products became safer as tighter screening methods were implemented and advanced modes of viral inactivation were utilized. In addition, synthetic (not derived from plasma) factor products were manufactured using recombinant technologies. In 1992, the first recombinant factor VIII product was approved by the Food and Drug Administration (FDA). In 1997, the first factor IX product was granted FDA approval.

By the mid-1990s, prophylactic (a preventative treatment regimen) therapy in children with hemophilia became more common. Proponents argued that the implementation of prophylaxis would prevent the chronic bleeding episodes that typically characterized hemophilia. Since the advent of prophylaxis, children could look forward to a life of less pain, without the orthopedic damage associated with chronic bleeding. As a result, most children born with hemophilia in the United States today can look forward to long, healthy, and active lives.

*Courtesy of the National Hemophilia Foundation, 2007

I think my mother certainly did the best she could with the situation. I don't think she anguished over it, but I think, as with everything, she put her whole self into it and did all she could.

Bob Jarratt

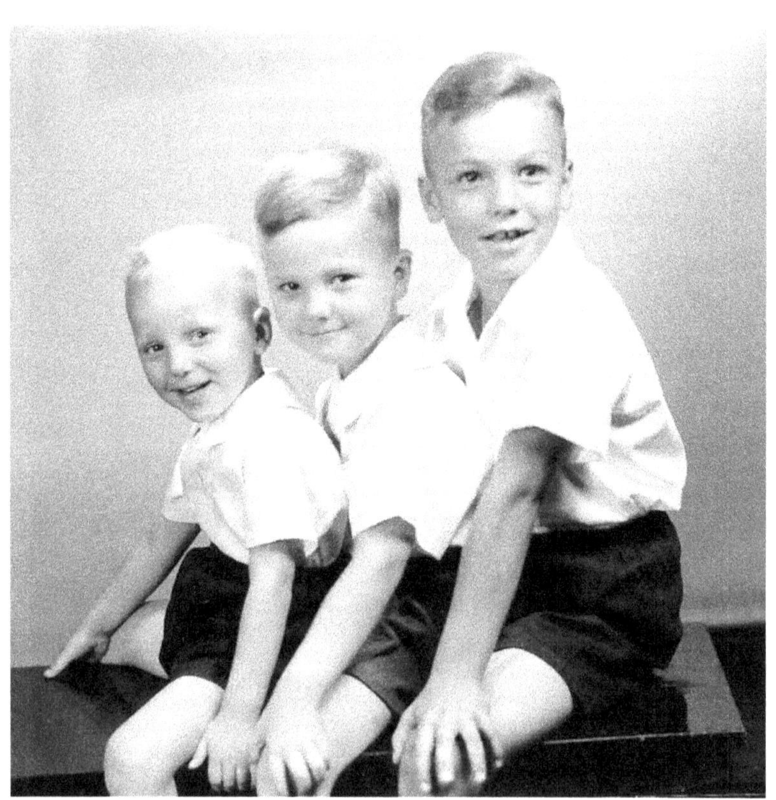

John, Jim and Bob Jarratt.

BOB JARRATT

Mr. Robert Jarratt was born in 1943 in Tennessee. He is married and has a daughter. Bob was diagnosed when he was in the Air Force and the confirmation of his diagnosis ended his military career. After open-heart surgery in the mid-1990s, Mr. Jarratt volunteered for the New England Hemophilia Association because he wanted to give something back in recognition of all the support and care he received from the hemophilia community. He has moderate factor IX deficiency.

They discovered that my brother, Jim, had a factor IX deficiency. When I came home on leave, our family doctor checked me and found that I also had factor IX deficiency. I went back to the Air Force and let them know about it. They ran their own tests and one of the tests produced a hematoma in my arm. They decided that they really didn't want any part of me, so they let me out of the service.

The head of the group I was in spoke to me as I left and said he was sorry that it had to work out this way. He wished me the best and sent me on my way.

It was not as though there was any choice on my part. The hematologist at Vanderbilt wrote to the Air Force to say that I wanted to be assigned to a job in a location where I could get reasonable medical care. The Air Force responded that they could not always guarantee that, so they got me out.

My mother, Gracie Faye, wasn't college-educated, but she began taking courses, through the Great Books. She read everything she could get her hands on and was probably the most well-educated person I have ever known. She went after information wholeheartedly. She became as knowledgeable as she could about hemophilia and was probably better informed than most of the doctors she ran into, not the specialists, but the general practitioners.

We were very lucky to have her.

I think my mother certainly did the best she could with the situation. I don't think she anguished over it, but I think, as with everything, she put her whole self into it and did all she could.

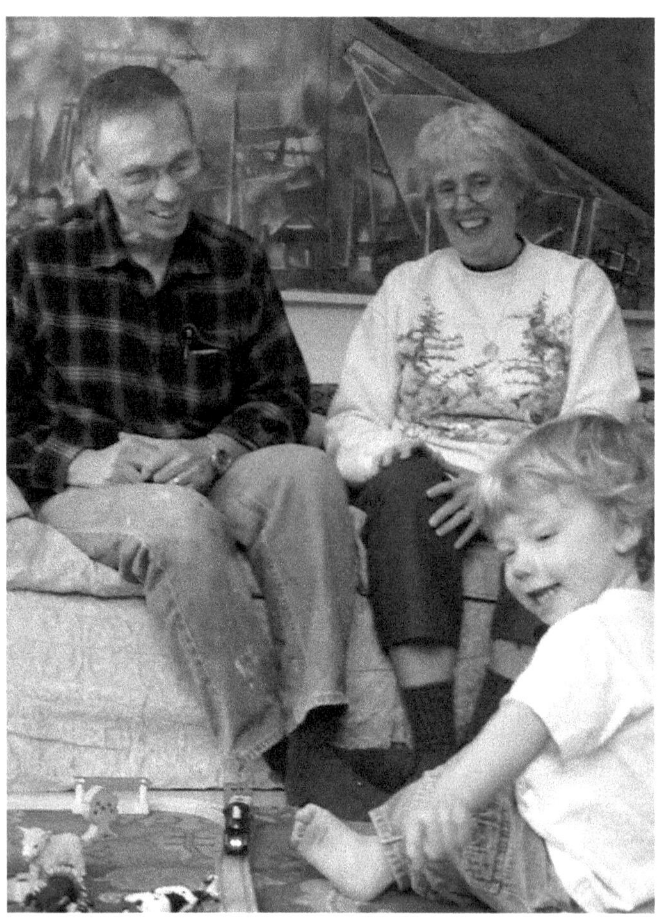

Bob and Claudia with their grandson, Benjamin.

I should also say that we're pretty certain now that Mom was also affected by the hemophilia, even though at the time people said that was not true for women. They realize now that, indeed, women can be affected. I don't know any real incidents, but she told us that she felt she also was affected by this. For example, she was anemic.

One of the general screening tests my cardiologist ran, an echocardiogram, indicated that I had a bicuspid aortic valve.

"You know," he said, "you just need to watch this as time goes on because they're more prone to calcify than others." That was pretty much it. They ran more tests and found that, indeed, the valve wasn't working properly and that there was an aneurysm around the aorta.

"We need to schedule surgery pretty quickly," the doctor told me, "and in the meantime, don't exert yourself. Don't lift anything."

My wife Claudia pointed out that I couldn't be operated on like this.

"It will be fine," the doctor said. "They'll work it out."

The doctor was right in that it certainly worked out, but there were issues that I think he wasn't truly aware of. Claudia got on the phone with the New England Hemophilia Society, talked to Cathy Cornell there and everything was pretty well set up for me. They got me into the hospital the day before and started giving me factor. Just before the surgery, they took some of my blood to give back to me after the surgery. They were really on top of it all the way.

I asked about the lifetime of the valve they were going to put in and my cardiologist answered, "Well, they can last a lifetime."

I was afraid. I think the most depressing moment came when they told me that they couldn't use the artificial valve because of my hemophilia – that type of valve requires the use of blood thinners. That meant that at some point I'd have to do it all again. I had to have a different type of valve, one that didn't have an unlimited lifetime. That, to me, was the most discouraging part.

It's not as though there was a choice, you know. If I have to do it again, I have to do it again. That procedure represented an astounding advance because certainly twenty — maybe even fifteen — years ago, I wouldn't have lived through that surgery.

After my surgery I was deeply aware of how caring the hemophilia community is – the doctors I met, Cathy and the people at the Hemophilia Treatment Center, the homecare people that we had. I wanted to do something, so I contacted Cathy and pretty much since then I've been involved with their newsletter committee.

I always brought up the fact that I was a hemophiliac when applying for jobs. I guess I was afraid not to, afraid of the consequences more than I was afraid of facing the problem up front. Fortunately, it wasn't an issue with anyone I worked with.

Brenda Nielsen and Aime Grimsley are nurses in the University of North Carolina at Chapel Hill Comprehensive Hemophilia Treatment Center. Both Brenda and Aime have treated patients with hemophilia since the 1980s.

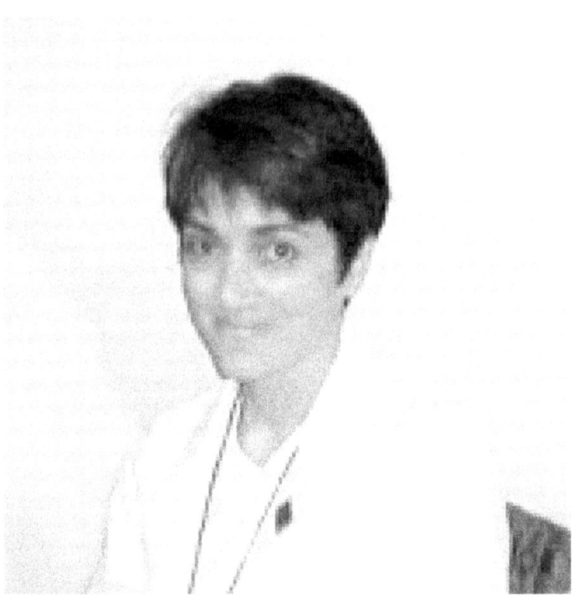

Aime Grimsley

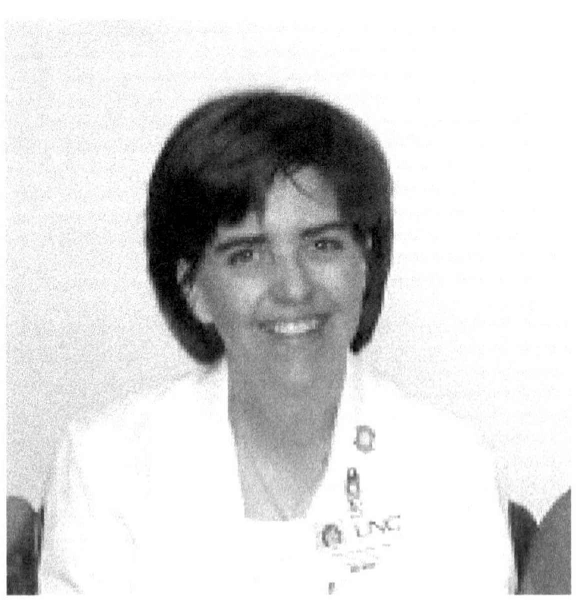

Brenda Nielsen

BRENDA NIELSEN AND AIME GRIMSLEY

Brenda Nielsen and Aime Grimsley are nurses in the University of North Carolina at Chapel Hill Comprehensive Hemophilia Treatment Center. Both Brenda and Aime have treated patients with hemophilia since the 1980s.

Aime

I wanted to work with the hemophilia patients because it was emotionally and intellectually challenging. You really do get to know patients and their families very well. You develop a closeness with your patients that you don't necessarily have with people who have another chronic illness, like diabetes or heart disease, because the hemophilia patients were, at the time, stigmatized. People were afraid. There were a lot of nurses, even then, who wouldn't take care of people with HIV.

In 1983, the life expectancy was two years if you were infected with HIV. We lost a few patients right off the bat, very early on but, for the most part, people were healthy. There was a lot of uncertainty, even on the part of the physicians, about what the positive test results meant. The hope was that a positive test meant that a person had only been exposed to HIV. It wasn't clear for a long time that it meant you were going to get sick.

Aime

Many people were very stoic, and kept the positive diagnosis to themselves. There were other people who were very well-connected in their community and open with their families and spouses, and everybody knew. We had some people who, after years of not telling, decided to share their HIV status because they needed support and ended up being kicked out of their churches and ostracized.

No one was given AZT until they had an infection. By that time, the patients were really sick and dying quickly. In those days, we would have maybe nine people die a year. It was really hard. We set up the home health, we set up the hospice, we were on the phone with the caregivers every day. At that time, there was a big stigma about going into the Infectious Disease Clinic, so we were it.

Brenda

A lot of the mothers were wrecks — emotional, physical wrecks. They are still devastated. We still talk to a lot of the parents. Their kids died six, seven, eight, ten years ago and we still talk to the parents. They call.

Aime

People moved here for treatment because early on we had a home infusion program, very early clotting concentrates, and very early treatment for inhibitors. Parents were doing what they thought was the best possible thing for their kids, and they were, but it had a bad outcome.

Aime

One person was ugly and yelled, "You all murdered my grandson!" That was hurtful, because I liked her grandson. It was hard to hear, but she needed to say it, and it was okay. I knew I hadn't murdered her grandson.

Brenda

You can't be with someone as they're dying and not sense that the spirit of that person, the life of that person, is still there. I mean, you can feel someone's spirit leave! I think it definitely deepens your sense of place and connection, the sense that people come into your life for a reason at different times. We're really all gifts to one another.

I think we all thought we had HIV. We would think back to our needle sticks and exposures, panic and think, "No, I've got it." You had this fantasy worry that you had contracted HIV. In those days, it was so prevalent in your mind that sometimes it would show up in your dreams.

Aime

There are women now who remember what their fathers dealt with.

"Daddy would stay in bed for two weeks, and when he'd scream all night in pain, Mama would call the doctor. He'd come put morphine in dad's arm, then he'd be okay."

The women talk a lot about those memories, and it takes a lot to convince them that they can expect something different for their child today. Hemophilia is still not easy, but it's a lot more manageable.

Aime

The hemophilia community is really special. The men are incredibly strong. The families are incredibly strong. Now, many of the men are moving into older age. Not long ago, people didn't live to be sixty, seventy — that was unusual. Now they're living longer and dealing with all the chronic illnesses like prostate cancer! No one with hemophilia got prostate cancer back in the seventies because no one lived that long!

I hear some men say, "I lived long enough to get prostate cancer!"

Love, that's what matters.

David LePage

DAVID LEPAGE

Mr. David LePage was born in 1963. David, who is single and lives alone, has dealt with mental and physical challenges throughout his life. He has been a public speaker about his experiences as a person living with chronic illness, and has found that his faith has been an enormous support. David has severe factor VIII deficiency, HIV and was successfully treated for hepatitis C.

When I was a teenager, I fought my parents because I wanted to take karate, but every time I blocked a punch, I would swell up. That was discouraging because I wanted to be a Black Belt. I wanted to be able to protect my faith, to protect myself against the world, and hemophilia was a big obstacle.

Because I would go to school on crutches one day and the next day I would be walking on my own, the kids would say I was faking. They didn't understand the disease of hemophilia, that you could be on crutches one day and not on crutches the next.

They tested me for HIV and a week later, they gave me the results. I was practically crying. Finding out that I had HIV rattled my father's cage; my uncles and aunts were shocked; my sister was terrified; but they were all very supportive.

I was sad and devastated when I found out, in particular knowing that chances for a girlfriend were difficult, but I couldn't let that affect me as a person.

I was living in a one-bedroom apartment when I was diagnosed. At that point, I wasn't afraid to tell anybody about the HIV or its complications, so I told my landlord. They forced me out of the apartment.

I found another apartment, and by then I had learned not to tell my landlord. I learned that honesty wasn't always the best policy.

I wish in many ways that my healthcare providers had been more supportive. That means taking a more active part in my life, calling me once in a while to see how I'm doing, so that I feel that they really care. I am passive in terms of my care, but I can also be assertive. Generally, I don't ask too much of my providers; I just go with the flow.

~

Just taking care of myself each day is enough of a fulfillment for me.

I don't have a lot of special interests or goals beyond just being able to try to live a normal life, a life with which I'm happy. Having a relationship here and there with somebody special makes life a lot easier.

I told my nurse that I had found somebody special and she said to me, "Well, David, you're special, too."

~

The pharmaceutical companies, four of them in all, gave each hemophiliac a hundred thousand dollars. It's a small payment. I feel like I deserve five hundred million and that would just take care of all my needs the rest of my life. I received a hundred thousand dollars in January of 1998, and the government offered another hundred thousand for failing to protect the blood supply for hemophiliacs and others who received transfusions.

I've enjoyed the money. I appreciate the compensation they gave because it makes my life a little easier: I can eat a little better, take care of myself a little better, I can pay for my medications a little better. I was more than happy to accept it.

I go to a support group in Brockton for hemophiliacs who have HIV. A large portion of the survivors were there when I started the support group. Now, there are about two or three left, and I'm one of them.

They call me a miracle because I'm still alive.

~

I became a Born Again Christian in 1982, and for twenty-two years, I've read the Bible every day. My faith has helped me through the difficult times with hemophilia, HIV and hepatitis.

I'm more content now that I'm a Christian. Instead of being angry and bitter and having fits of rage over my illnesses, I try to be peaceable and gentle and take care about other people. It's a tough, tough thing to juggle. I'm not employed because of my mental disability, and I have all I can handle to manage all my diseases without working.

~

Trials in life produce character and encourage perseverance. Perseverance, character, and I still have hope.

And love, that's what matters.

Initially, we went to Boston every time I needed to be infused and that was a long way. But, you know, my folks took me and my father said to me one day — I'll never forget it — he said, 'I'd walk to China for you.'

Billy Lynch

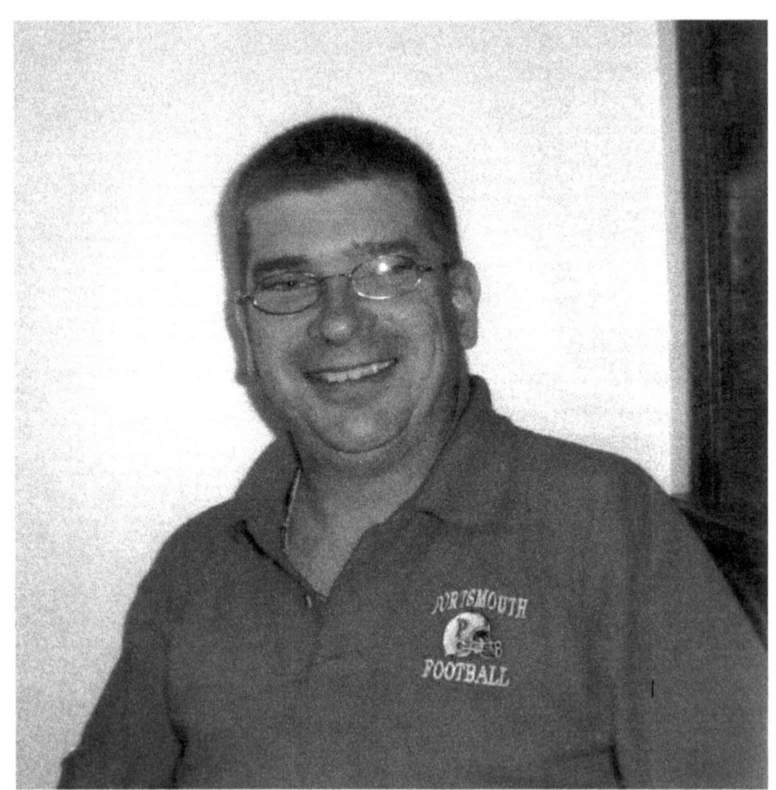

Billy Lynch at work.

BILLY LYNCH

Mr. William Lynch was born in 1960 in Fall River, Massachusetts. He went to school in Fall River; his mother was a nurse and his father was a school principal. When he was diagnosed with hemophilia at age one, it came as a surprise to his family because there was no history. He has two brothers, neither of whom has the disease. Billy attended Bridgewater State College, is single and works with the retarded.

He feels that factor manufacturers should have admitted that they made mistakes. He feels lucky to be alive and healthy and would never have imagined that he'd be this well in 2005. Billy has severe factor VIII, HIV and hepatitis C.

As a child, I was playing baseball and I got hit in the mouth. It had happened a few times earlier and I went to the hospital, but this was the one occasion that was tough. I had to go to the hospital and even at that age — I might have been ten, maybe a little younger — when it really hit. "Man, I've got a problem here."

It was like, "Hey, I'm sick of this already," and I was only a kid.

You're very angry at that point because you know you can't do all the things you did before. You look around at your brothers and your friends, at all your classmates, and you don't see anything wrong with them, so you think to yourself, "Why me, here?"

Initially we went to Boston every time I needed to be infused and that was a long way. But, you know, my folks took me and my father said to me one day, I'll never forget it, he said, "I'd walk to China for you."

When I got a little older, I realized that my parents were going through what I was going through, but when you're very young, you don't realize that. You think you're it. As I got older, I realized that when they were taking me to the hospital, all the time, they were suffering as much as I was.

Once I knew I couldn't do sports, I played the trumpet. I started that in the fourth grade and I pretty much stopped in my senior year in high school. To be truly honest with you, when I look back, the trumpet was an alternative to athletics, but I still would have taken the sports, although I wouldn't have gone anywhere. One, I was too short. Two, I just wasn't good enough, but at least I would have been out there trying.

The trumpet was a good alternative. I played in the high school band, and it was okay. I look back with fond memories, but at the time, my heart wasn't in it. I was also a scorer for the middle school basketball team. You're in the locker room before the game and you want to be on that team, but I did what I could and I did a nice job scoring. And I got to see all the games.

As a child you're angry. God or no God, you're very angry. When I got older, I became aware of other sick people for the first time, and that helped me handle my own problems. When I went to Children's Hospital in the early '80s, when I was about twenty-one, to have my wisdom teeth out, I saw a lot of kids suffering, with IV's, with bald heads, and that experience transformed me.

I said to myself, "Man, what are you — you're lucky," and I really have had that attitude since then. The "Why mes?" kind of stopped. That's when I really started counting my blessings.

Suddenly you look around at other people who are dealing with worse situations than you are, whereas, as a kid, most people you see are fine.

I was born with something that was totally out of my control, but as I look back, I think it has made me more compassionate. It has definitely made me more understanding. Professionally I have worked twenty-one years with the mentally retarded. They don't have hemophilia, but they have problems, and I have compassion for that.

As I look back, I think my experience has made me a better person as an adult.

The naturally kind people, the ones who have the big hearts, I think they can more or less understand everything. You could have cancer, hemophilia or a bad case of diabetes, and I think they have an understanding. The average person, no. Most people wouldn't know what it's like to have a particular disease.

We're Catholic and, thankfully, they brought me up in the Catholic faith, very strongly. That has a lot to do with how I dealt with the ramifications of the hemophilia. Number one to me is my faith. I give credit to my folks right from the get-go.

I wouldn't take away my senior year of college for anything. More than thirty of us went to Jacksonville, Florida in two vans. Oh, it was living hell for me to drive that far, but we had a great time when we got down there.

I did have one bleed on that trip. No big deal, but I went to mix the factor and it had expired. The local hospitals didn't have any factor, so three of us went to Jacksonville where they had the factor. It took a couple of hours, but it wasn't bad. The woman and the guy who made the trip with me were very, very happy. We were listening to the radio blaring as we drove to the hospital.

It has happened quite a bit throughout my years, the times when you say, "Oh, why now?" You deal with it the best you can and try to get to the factor the best you can and that's that. The problem with hemophilia and other disabilities is that you don't always have answers, so you pretty much have to meet it head on and go for it.

Actually, there were different pains. You had the arthritis pain, which was a very sharp pain: sometimes, it got to the point where it was agonizing. You had to sit down. The bleed is a different type of pain. It's pressure, but it got to the point where it was unbearable. If you had a bleed that you couldn't get to right away, it was unbearable.

It's funny, though, you adjust to it. As difficult as it is, you adjust to it.

Hemophilia.

I don't like the word sometimes, you know.

Accommodation came over a period of time. I didn't sit down one day and say, "Bang, I'm grateful." You know, "Bang, I can deal with it." I think it was little by little. It was a lifelong experience to come to this point; it wasn't anything automatic. I got a little smarter, I think, as I got older.

I have hepatitis C, and the last few years I've had blood work every three or four months. They wanted a liver biopsy and I told them, "No. I'll go on interferon. I have no problem, but I'm not going to go for a biopsy right now."

What can they do? So they find out fifty percent of the liver is damaged. Medically, what can they do? Nothing. So I thought, I'll deal with the iffy.

It allows me to remain hopeful. I know what could happen, but I don't have to live with it every day. You've got a life out there you have to live, and the possibility is always in the back of your mind, but I felt a biopsy was going to bring it to the forefront.

The HIV crisis was even more of a concern than the hepatitis C, so back in 1985, I said, "All right, test me."

They never called me with the results. Never called me, positive, negative. No one called me back, and you don't know what to think of that. We looked at the file years later and all the record showed was that I had been tested. They didn't have the results. All hell was breaking loose and, as time went on, I refused to be tested again. I stayed away from the hemophilia clinic.

I let them do a T-cell count in May of '91, and the numbers had gone down. I knew what the problem was at that point, you know what I mean? So I said, "Test me."

It was awful because I knew what it was. Back then, they had nothing. They had the AZT and that was really about it. My mother and father both have so much faith, and my father, I think — and he never told me this, it's just my gut feeling — I think he had hoped like hell that maybe I was one of those five percent that tested negative.

He cried on the way home. I was numb. That was the word, numb, because it wasn't unexpected. That was thirteen years ago.

Financially, I shouldn't have a worry in the world, but I commend the people who worked so hard for the settlement. I commend them. The word thank you doesn't describe it, that's how grateful I am to them. They did the best they could. I guess if I had gone it alone, I probably would have lost. So I think they did the best they could, but it will never be over, in my opinion, until the drug companies actually say, "We made a mistake. We were wrong."

I mean, why would you give a hundred thousand dollars to every hemophiliac, I don't know how many hundred million, and not actually say, "we're guilty"? They should have admitted guilt, and they never did, as far as I know.

I have a Bachelor's in history, and now I'm going for an Associate's degree in Business. I have a chance at the company where my brother works and I have several references, so I think I could get in, but I'm worried about insurance. With hemophilia, you need the insurance and I feel trapped sometimes.

And then I worry if, when they find out about my medical record, would they say, "Sorry, we can't cover this guy?"

I'm afraid of the insurance and the HIV and the hepatitis. All I need is to leave my job and have the next employer say, "We can't do it." That happened once in the early '80s, and it broke my heart. All it was was sorting newspapers. That's all it was, but I thought, "Just get in there," maybe I could become a sports reporter or a journalist.

Well, before I started, I went for a physical. Often back then they were kind of amazed by hemophiliacs. So I went for a physical and I passed. I didn't get any calls, so I called them back. I didn't hear anything. Well, it was the hemophilia, that's why they didn't hire me for that job and it was because they were afraid, in case something happened to me. God, was I mad, and, even though it was a long time ago, I'm afraid something like that might happen again.

It's like life insurance. I can't get life insurance except through the State. They just had an open enrollment for the State and I grabbed the whole thing. I grabbed as much as I could. If you work for the State, they will give it to you, no questions asked.

That's very restricting for me as a person. It's terrible, to be honest with you. I can't leave the job because of my insurance. I'm trapped.

You want to know something, though? I started working young; when I was fourteen I was doing painting. It was part of what they called the Youth Resource Agency. They were very nice to me, those people, and they hired me. I worked at the Venus DeMilo, a fancy restaurant in Swansea, Massachusetts, that does weddings and a lot of big banquets. They hired me. The only thing the owner said to me was, "Just watch out for broken glass."

If I ever saw them again, I'd tell them how much that meant to me. I really would.

I've been the kind of a guy who has a date here and there. I've never really been at the point where I wanted to get married. Do I think the disease has something to do with it? Would I get married? Absolutely, but you'd need somebody real, real special, because who wants to marry somebody with HIV and hepatitis C? Now, I know there are exceptions out there, but, to me, what a tough thing. I've never really met any women yet who are in that category.

I've never been so close to a woman that I've had to tell her. I might deny

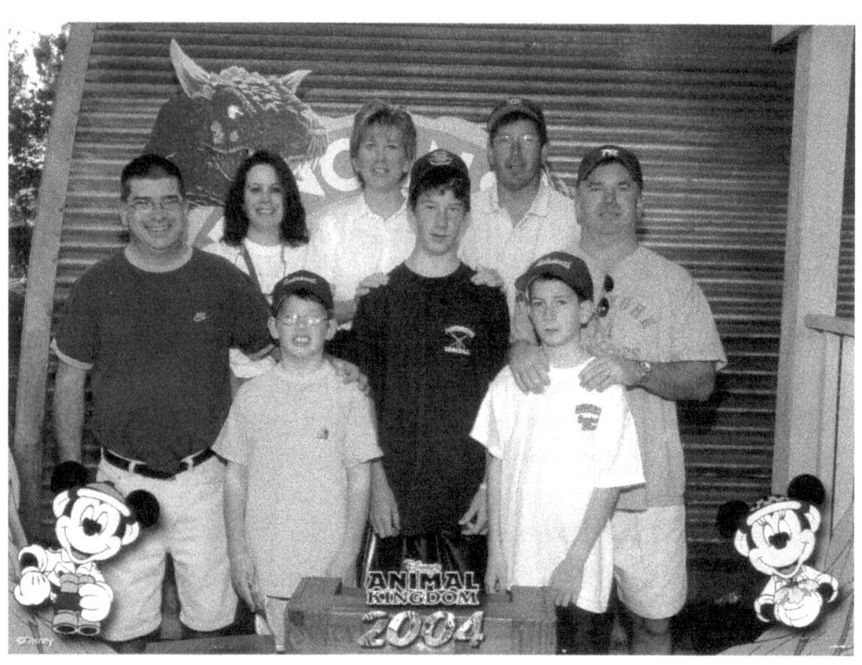

Billy in Florida with his brothers, sisters-in-law and nephews.

it, but I really think that what is preventing me from developing a relationship is that I don't want to put myself in that position, where I have to tell someone, "Geez, I have hemophilia." It's a big-time threat.

You're avoiding a huge problem if you don't get close to anyone.

Actually, my knees are much better. Having them replaced was the best thing I ever did. I had them done three years apart, and it was a lot of hard work and physical therapy, and I worked my tail off both times. I have more muscle tone now and I'm walking three miles every other day now.

It wasn't a hard decision. I had had it. I was in pain all the time. I walked terribly and I held out until my late thirties, so I did all right. I was healthy, so they did the surgery. I do have a problem with my elbow occasionally, but nothing compared to what these knees were.

I think if I had a chance to do things again, in my younger years I would have chosen to have been less bitter.

There were times when I was angry because I couldn't play certain sports. Like one time I was playing football. No, no, I was stupid, okay, I'll admit it. I was playing a position where there wasn't much contact, and I had pads on, but my father came down and took me out. Oh, was I mad!

Back then you're incredibly mad, but now I understand.

I talked about it with my parents, but they didn't have the answers. No one has the answers. Like most good parents do, they tried to get me to enjoy something else, to teach me to be moderate.

Let's say you have somebody with hemophilia, someone who's fourteen right now, and he's a gifted athlete. What I would tell him is, "Play hard." You can't go out there and not play hard, right? You really can't. Play hard but don't play stupid. If there's a ball that you know you're not going to get, don't dive for it.

But just to play, that's lousy. You want to go one hundred percent when you're playing those games, and I couldn't. I really couldn't.

I have definitely looked at mortality and looked at it a lot — to be honest with you, almost every day, I think about it. You think about it to the point where it doesn't really affect you. Over the last thirteen years, I've been trying to prepare myself to get sick. I'm lucky in that I have had that chance, that I didn't walk in there in '91 and find that I was near death at that point.

I consider myself very fortunate to have lived this long, to have been able to prepare myself. If I do get sick, I think I'm better prepared now than I would have been ten years ago. My faith has a lot to do with that, plus a lot of people whom you thought would outlive you because you had the HIV virus and they didn't, have died.

I am incredibly lucky to be healthy now because if you had told me in '91 that I'd still be healthy in 2004, I would have laughed at you. And here I am.

I think as far as death goes, for a guy forty-four, I'm handling it the best I can. In other words, it won't be a shocker. I've kind of been able to learn to take it one day at a time and knowing that, "Yeah, I might get sick," I look at it as though I'm preparing myself for that.

I think I've been pretty much at peace the last four years.

I'm used to the idea of HIV and hep C. My folks are used to it. My brothers are used to it. I think some of my friends don't even think about it anymore, because I've had it for so long. But I do wonder what other people, people who don't know about me right now, would think if they were told. They might go through the process I went through twelve years ago.

You just can't let the HIV thing get to you. You've got to accept it, and it's very difficult to accept it when you get it from blood, but you have to. The day you accept it, your life becomes a little easier.

My parents may have said "Be careful," but, thank God, they didn't say "Don't do this," or "Don't do that." Can you imagine a life like that? I would have been miserable.

Jack Rollins

JACK ROLLINS

Mr. Rollins was born in 1933 in Brighton, Massachusetts and has moderate factor IX deficiency. He is married and has two children. He is a certified public accountant and has worked all over the world.

He hasn't wanted to reveal his diagnosis since he was asked to leave Notre Dame a day after he arrived as a result of revealing that he had hemophilia.

When I was a kid, I was always fighting. It was either a sport or we got mad at each other, one or the other, and I always stopped the fight with my nosebleeds. Whack, and there was blood all over the place and that would call off the fight and I'd go home to try to stop my nosebleed.

My brother had a transfusion after he was in an automobile accident and that got him. He died. My cousin and my brother both got AIDS.

I got whacked from the side. My head hit a post and I started bleeding, unbeknownst to me, until a couple of days later. There was a bump and it got larger and larger and larger, and it wouldn't go down. As soon as everyone realized there was something wrong, they put me in the hospital and found an internist. Cortisone had just come out, and he tried treating me with that. I don't know whether it worked or not. Finally, they cut my head and just let everything out, and then put a bandage on.

Boy, did that thing hurt because of the big swelling.

They took me into the Ether Dome, where ether was first administered at Mass General Hospital. It's an amphitheater, and that's where they hold meetings. They rolled me down, "Hey, you're coming with us," and talked about me — Exhibit A.

They shaved my head, and that was the worst experience of my life.

I was accepted at Notre Dame University. I wasn't going to get into football games or basketball games there, rough games, because I didn't want to get whacked again. So I brought a letter with me and after a couple of days I took it down. The letter said that I was a hemophiliac. I showed them the letter and the next day I was on a train back home. They didn't want to take a chance with me.

From that day forward, I never told a soul that I had hemophilia. I didn't want to tell my employer that I had this problem. I didn't want the insurance company to know that I had the problem, or anyone else. I decided I would pay for things myself.

I was playing baseball and I was the catcher, which wasn't the smartest thing in the world. There was no equipment; I had a glove and that was about it. A guy came piling in from third base and whacked me on the head.

I decided I wouldn't play catcher any more. There were certain things that I was going to avoid.

When I was twenty-two, I took a four-month bicycle/motorcycle trip in Europe and I wore a helmet as a concession to my parents. They bought me a helmet and told me to wear it. People didn't wear helmets in those days, you know, not for anything.

My parents may have said "Be careful," but, thank God my parents didn't say "Don't do this," or "Don't do that." Can you imagine a life like that? I would have been miserable.

I'm not too sure I'd want to tell my kids not to do something. I think if they came up short — got whacked over the head with a baseball bat, for example — and it proved serious, then they would know on their own and would have learned a lesson.

They tried to keep the HIV testing 'anonymous,' which is sort of a joke. They assigned you a test number and this employee from the Department of Health said, "I'll meet you somewhere and give you the news." He met me in the parking lot of a local department store. I rolled down my window and he rolled down his and he said, "You're positive. Have a nice day."

Mike Dowling

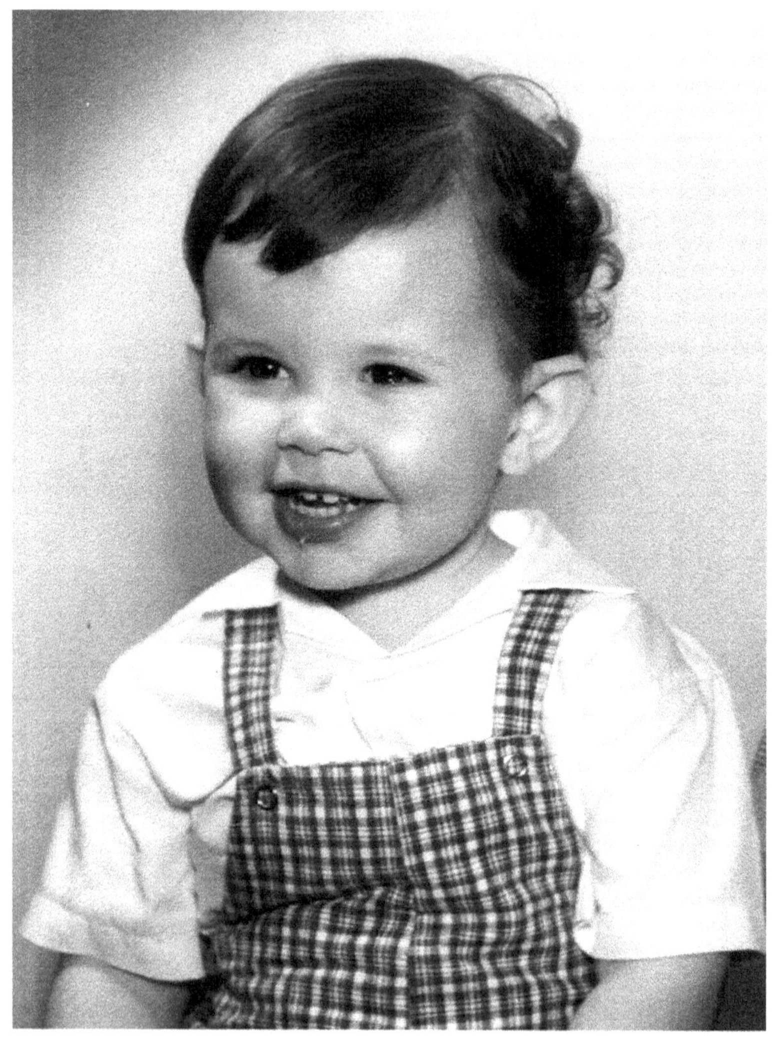

Mikey

MIKE DOWLING

Mr. Michael Dowling was born in 1960 and raised in a small town in northwestern Vermont. There was no family history of hemophilia and his brother, three years younger, was not affected. Michael attended college in Vermont and later became involved in statewide groups addressing issues of concern to the HIV community.

Mike was diagnosed as an infant with severe factor VIII deficiency and has HIV and hepatitis C.

One of my earlier memories of hemophilia was a fairly major bleed that I incurred. We were over in Maine on vacation when I was about five and I fell off the back of a picnic table and landed on my head. That night in the hotel, I started having nosebleeds. My eyes were looking in opposite directions. The left eye was looking left and the right eye was looking right, so the vision was no longer coordinated and I had headaches. My folks didn't have any resources in rural Maine, so we packed up everything, left the motel room that night and drove straight back to Burlington.

I was in the hospital with severe concussion and a lot of hemorrhaging inside the head and the brain. I didn't know anybody and I didn't even recognize my own folks. I have few early childhood memories from before that because that incident kind of wiped the slate clean for me. I was in the hospital for a long period of time, six weeks, and the nurses shaved all my hair off. They had wires coming out of my head where they were doing brain scans and things like that; gradually, they encouraged relatives and friends, trying to jog my memory.

When I got out of the hospital, there were a bunch of changes in my life as a result. I had been skinny as a young child, and now I gained all kinds of weight. I had an insatiable hunger when I was in the hospital. I wanted to eat all the time, and the doctors, knowing I was quite sick, actually encouraged me. I ballooned, I mean, I got heavy in a hurry, both in the hospital, as well as out. Once I got out of the hospital, I gained weight that basically stuck with me for most of my life. I only ended up at five foot four, so I'm not a tall man. I've basically been below average most of my life, height-wise.

I wore a blue baseball helmet, which became my moniker. Doctors recommended it: they said "Maybe next time he won't be that fortunate." So I had a baseball helmet that I wore any time I went outside the house. It certainly set me apart from most of the other kids and I kind of became known for it.

I was out playing basketball one day with a friend, just shooting hoops, and the ball ricocheted off the basket and took the visor part of the helmet right off. All I had left was this hard plastic beanie. We tried to glue the visor back on, but it wasn't going to stay. Then they fitted me for a construction helmet, but it was an adult construction helmet, one of those big yellow hardhat things, and the thing stuck out several inches around my whole head. It was massive. There was no way.

I wore that for a short period of time and said, "Forget it. I've had enough."

I got some good years out of that blue helmet. Everybody knew me by my helmet. I guess it made me feel safer, not that I really expected to have something drop out of the sky on me, anyway.

I was in a little four-room schoolhouse with first and second grade downstairs and third and fourth upstairs, a few blocks from where I grew up. Crutches certainly were fairly common when I was in elementary school, but there were challenges. The schools were not handicapped-accessible, so just getting upstairs was sometimes a challenge. There were no elevators or anything like that back then.

My condition was certainly very painful and there weren't an awful lot of options at the time for the treatment of pain. I don't think they wanted to get into narcotics, particularly with a child. I would take aspirin by the bottle, not knowing that it was actually making the pain worse. Back in the '60s they didn't have any other options; they knew nothing about Tylenol or about the bleeding side-effects of aspirin.

My father would come in quite often and rub my joints with rubbing alcohol. It felt cool to the joints; his soft touch and his being there was certainly very beneficial. The pain was a fact of life, just something I had to endure.

My father has a good sense of humor and he's always very upbeat. My mother is kind of nervous and high-strung and wasn't perhaps as good at dealing with some of the medical issues as my father was. She, like some other moms, would tend to get more emotional, while he would stay more level-headed. "All right," he'd say, "we'll deal with this," and "Let's find out what we can do and if we need tests done." My father was certainly much more proactive in staying calm and getting things done. That was reassuring. It felt as though he was taking action, even though there wasn't always a lot he could do.

My bedroom was upstairs, and my father used to carry me on his back because it was hard to navigate stairs with crutches. If you had two things going on simulta-neously, if you were having an elbow bleed at the same time you were having a knee bleed, it made it a real challenge. I would latch onto him and he'd carry me upstairs, even when I weighed way over a hundred pounds.

The other problem they had back in the '60s was cross-matching the blood, and sometimes you'd get a bad pint. It just plain hadn't been cross-matched well enough, and when that happened, you usually knew fairly quickly because you'd break out in hives and get sweaty. They knew right away what to do; they obviously stopped that transfusion and hung a different bottle of blood, or flushed the lines. There wasn't an awful lot they could do to reverse the effects; those just sort of went away on their own.

Life was sometimes put on hold for the family. I delayed trips. It wasn't like we didn't make plans, but the plans were derailed sometimes as a result of my condition. I felt bad because I was the cause. If we were scheduled to go to Maine on vacation and I came down with a giant bleed just before we were due to go, it was obviously disappointing to my folks, to myself and to my brother. But my brother was great, and he never said anything. I look back on it now and I wonder if maybe he resented it, because I certainly got an awful lot more attention than he ever got as a child.

I don't recall being teased an awful lot. There was one kind of tough kid when I got into junior high school who I remember running across a few times. In the hall, he'd say, "Hey, hemo." That was his nickname for me, and I didn't like it.

In general, I liked the kids and I think the kids liked me. In high school, getting involved with the music program, both the chorus and the band, gave me a reason not to rush right home after school. Typically, the practices and rehearsals were in the evening, so it gave me a sense of independence to be there. By my junior year I had my license, and my parents would let me use the car, which gave me even more independence and probably gave my mother more gray hairs.

❧

By the time I was a teenager, we had cryoprecipitate and fresh frozen plasma and the transfusions could be done a lot faster. I had to go to the hospital to have transfusions done, but I could have it done right in the ER or outpatient, which at that particular hospital were basically the same thing. That allowed more independence and far fewer hospitalizations.

❧

For most of my life, I was the only person in town with hemophilia, so there wasn't anybody really networkable for my folks or for myself.

Even finding babysitters was a challenge for my folks, because there wasn't a plethora of teenage girls out there who were willing to take on the responsibility for somebody who had special needs. They would say no.

❧

A lot of times I'd wake up with pain. You'd be up and about and watching TV and your folks were there and there was noise and lights and smells and distractions. Then you would be alone in bed in a dark, quiet room and it was just you and pain.

❧

A young pediatrician came to town, fairly fresh out of med school. My other pedia-trician, whom I'd had for probably the first ten years or so, had died of a heart attack. This young doctor certainly had a familiarity with hemophilia and was willing to take on the case and do some research into it. He knew what they were doing in other areas of the country and he was a little more progressive about treatment options for me.

This new physician said to my father, who was often more present in my healthcare than my mother was, "Perhaps he could learn how to do home infusion." It was not being done in the state of Vermont and I don't think it was even being done in northern New England at that time. So we looked into the possibility of keeping the medicine in my fridge, having my father mix it and then having him start an IV. There was certainly a training issue for my father, although he had seen it done a thousand times because he was there by the bedside. He knew that, in terms of my healthcare, it would improve things greatly and give me more independence.

Looking back, knowing that it was probably going to take half a dozen stabs for the pros to do it, it was like, "Hey, Dad, give it a shot. You can't do any worse than the doctors are doing!" We took the old slide projector screen — if you recall, they had a pole with a hook on the top for the screen — and we'd hang the bottles from that for the drip. We had to improvise back then.

My mother couldn't even be in the room. My father stepped up and accepted that responsibility, so it didn't bother me that she couldn't. There were times when I knew I was having a bleed and if he was local and it was convenient, he would swing home and do it. Other times, it would just be a matter of waiting until he got home, but I'd rather do that than go to the hospital.

There were some battles that we had to fight, first off with the insurance company. The insurance company said they weren't going to cover the high expense of the medicine or accept the risk or responsibility of having it done outside a hospital setting.

Certainly the amount of medicine I was taking with factor concentrate was considerably smaller. I didn't get that bloated feeling and it worked much better. Even when I was a kid, I knew that there was only a drop or two in that pint of blood that I was slowly watching drip into me that was doing me any good. The rest of it was added fluid. They just didn't have the technology to be able to extract that drop or two that was really beneficial. With the factor, if you caught a bleed fairly early, you could eliminate a lot of the pain and swelling and you were more mobile faster.

They talked a lot about developing an aura when you were bleeding, so that you would catch it early. I had problems identifying that aura initially, being able to diagnose my own body when something was going wrong. It wasn't something they could teach you to do.

I know some of the warning signs when things are just not right. You either start to feel a twinge or a pain or maybe you just can't straighten that elbow out quite as well as you thought you could before, or the knee seems to be boggy, and there's a different kind of pain than you experience from arthritis. You have to be able to differentiate. I don't want to cry foul and run and infuse every time I'm a little stiff getting out of a chair, but I also need to be aware.

In the morning, I do a kind of self-diagnostic check-up myself. I would typically wake up in the morning with a bleed. Probably something had been festering the night before, but when I went to bed, I didn't pick up the warning signs. Then I was sedentary for six or eight or more hours and when I woke up, I couldn't move my elbow or I couldn't move my ankle. By that time, it's almost too late. You're tired and it's late and it's like, "Ah, I'll do the wait-and-see attitude. Maybe it will be better tomorrow. Maybe it's just because I'm tired and I've had a physical day." You just don't want to bother. It's eleven o'clock at night. It's harder to find veins at that time of night, you know. You're tired, so you postpone it.

Backing up a little to high school, there was a family that moved into town with a son my age who had severe factor VIII hemophilia and he had inhibitors. He had gone through many of the same challenges I had, so we became friends in high school. We were also roommates in college.

He resented his folks. He resented having hemophilia. He was bitter about it and he was bitter towards his folks for even having him, knowing there was a chance that he could have hemophilia. I saw the darker side of things with him.

I found it interesting. I think if anything, it gave me more resolve to try to stay upbeat and chipper about things because I could see the other side. It was like, "Hey, that's not a side I want to be on."

I went to college in Vermont and there were some challenges. I didn't have a car when I started, so when I had a bleed, I went over to the local hospital. They're the largest medical center in the state, so they get all the critical cases. I'd either walk over or, more often than not, I'd get security to give me a ride over. It was not uncommon for me to wait there eight to ten hours for treatment. It took forever. I was going to keep the medicine in my own refrigerator and mix it, but gee, that wasn't practical when you might have to wait ten hours before they would infuse it.

Then I decided maybe I would try going through the school infirmary, which also wasn't that far physically from where I was. I could either walk down or they could give me a ride, particularly if I was having foot or leg challenges. They did okay. The shortcoming there was that they weren't open all the time, so you had to make sure you had your bleeds when it was convenient for them and not necessarily when it was convenient for you.

I've never had a lot of social life around females. I saw a gal through college. I was a little older and had a car, and I wined and dined her. We did things and went to concerts and sports events. I think a lot of the attraction for her was more what we did than really truly being in love with me. It was about having a good time. It sure beat sitting at home at night with her folks.

Love is finally part of my life now, but I didn't date in my twenties or thirties much at all. I decided that maybe it would be just too much for women to handle. That was probably true in high school, as well, and being way overweight didn't help. I was 5' 4" and 195 pounds. That doesn't give you an awful lot of self-confidence to go out there and ask women to go dating with you. It wasn't necessarily just the hemophilia. There were other things, too, but the hemophilia was certainly a drawback. There was a reluctance because I was different. I can't imagine most women, particularly high school kids, finding it desirable to see me when 99.9% of the rest of the population is "normal" and doesn't have that health problem. Why would they find me particularly attractive?

I've always been interested in sports. Even as a child, when I couldn't play Little League, I was an official scorer. I'd go down to the baseball park with the guys and hang out, report the scores back to the local paper, then go home to read my little report in our local newspaper.

You know, I was reading about HIV in the papers and it was kind of a horrifying thing because people were really getting sick. They were going blind and they were getting all these rare pneumonias. It was kind of scary.

By that time, there were hemophilia treatment centers and I was plugged into the one in Burlington, Vermont. I had a hematologist there who has long since retired, and a nurse practitioner who also has long since retired. The state got involved and they decided that since people with hemophilia were at a high risk, they would round us up and test us. So we weren't really asked if we wanted to be tested; we just were.

There were no consent forms or anything like that back then. The state just wanted to know who they had out there that had this.

I was in my early twenties at this point and I felt as though, yeah, there was a chance that it could be me. Knowing that I had taken a fairly high level of blood product through the years, I figured it out.

They tried to keep it "anonymous," which is sort of a joke. They assigned you a test number and this employee from the Department of Health said, "I'll meet you somewhere and give you the news." He met me in the parking lot of a local department store. I rolled down my window and he rolled down his and he said, "You're positive," then "Have a nice day."

There was no written literature or any back-up information about what that really meant. All I had was what I had been reading in the papers about these people. The thought crossed my mind, "Maybe I should just go jump off an interstate bridge somewhere, and save everybody a lot of pain and anguish here." I wasn't reading anything about people getting better, just about a lot of people who were getting really sick, really fast, and dying. So it wasn't exactly great news.

I can't say the diagnosis was completely shocking news to me. I was mentally kind of prepared for the possibility that this was going to be the case, and it was. I went into it prepared for the worst, rather than being naïve and saying, "Oh, there's no way that I could possibly have ever gotten it."

There was no real networking at all between the people with hemophilia. You'd come into clinic, but that would be about it. They'd whisk you off to a small examining room and you never really got an opportunity to meet any of the other people. There wasn't really the chance to network and there was no association or anything like that at the treatment center, or even outside the treatment center.

I didn't know what to expect and, really, neither did the medical industry. There weren't any drug treatments at all. They couldn't tell you what the probability was. They didn't have any scientific studies and they didn't even really have a lot of good information. There weren't a lot of published reports, other than in the newspapers, nothing scientific. And they didn't have a lot of good treatment options, so there wasn't much to do.

What you did realize early on was that there was a huge stigma around the whole issue of HIV. I knew I had to keep pretty tight-lipped about it, even though I was now working in a family business. I didn't tell any of the employees or coworkers at all. Disclosure became a big thing. I was old enough to realize that it had to be a guarded secret. That's true to a certain extent, even to this day, but I'm a lot more free-flowing with it now than I was then. You're not as much of an outcast now for having a blood disorder as you were then. There's a lot more understanding and many new treatment options.

I was aware of the discrimination issues early on, but I didn't think much at the time about the whole patient's rights thing and the way I was tested. I don't think anybody else did, either, even in the medical industry. It was like, "Oh, just take a blood test on him. We're doing blood tests all the time; just throw in an HIV test." It was just sort of matter of fact for the medical industry, and the whole idea of having permission or providing counseling or information never occurred to anybody in public health.

It wasn't until years later that I finally thought about it, that I opened my eyes, and it was like, "That's just not right, what they did."

That feeling may have fired up some inclination to become involved. How could I make a difference in the system, or feel as though I was? I was asked by someone from the state to join the Community Planning Group. They called five of us into a room; I had never met the other four. We were from representative communities that had been adversely affected by HIV. I was the token person with hemophilia.

The group was just getting started. They had received some funding through the CDC and it was a nationally-funded project designated to start these statewide organizations. It mandated that a large percentage of the group were to be consumers or patients, if you will, as opposed to health-care professionals. The question was, how could we come up with a plan for limiting the spread of HIV in the state?

I took this route instead of jumping off the bridge. I think it really was a positive thing for me, and it was good to know that there were a lot of other people out there who were really pulling hard to make a difference.

It was awkward for me in some respects to be that token person with hemophilia, because I had a good outlook on life. I had fairly good health, good support systems with my folks and good insurance. I grew up being a little naïve in a nice middle class family. To relate to somebody from the other end of the state who was economically disadvantaged and had a lot of challenges in his life, maybe from a broken family or a big family that didn't have health insurance and good access to health services in some rural area of the state, people who were not as well educated — not only did I not know them, but I felt somewhat awkward even speaking for them.

I was reassured that somebody has to, and that you can do it if you're sympathetic to the needs of those people and you know they're out there.

I knew one high school student who wasn't allowed to ride the bus. Things happened. The driver didn't want the responsibility and he wouldn't pick the child up. The hemophilia nurse coordinator had gone to bat for the family. They took it to court, which was a bold move even then because it exposes you. I guess the family felt they had nothing to lose because their status had been exposed already. The family, which was a rural family, sued and they started with the school. It went to the School Board. It went beyond the Board. They stuck by their guns and said, "Hey, if the bus driver doesn't want to pick him up, we side with him." It went through the courts.

I believe they determined that they did not need to pick up the child, that clearly the boy had something that was potentially unhealthy and potentially contagious.

So I knew about discrimination in the hemophilia population and I guess that bothered me. I knew the other side. I don't know if that's what spurred me on, but I felt as though somebody needed to be a spokesperson for this group, and I didn't know whether there was somebody else out there who was willing to step into my place to do that or not.

It was sort of a fluke that I started going out with a woman I had known for many years. She was from my home town originally and she's a few years older than I am. I sort of knew her from seeing her in church and we served together on a commission. I knew she was a single mom. Back a few years ago, we did a couple of things together. She knew I had been infected. Then I asked her outright around New Year's 2004 and we've been going out ever since.

She was quite an eye-opener to me about some of my health challenges and about my being absorbed in it. She could see that all I talked about was my health.

"You're a person first," she said, "and you need to remember that. Your priorities have gotten screwed up here. It's okay to be concerned about the health issues, but you live and breathe them. That's all you speak about — how you feel or the new medical study you've been reading about."

"You're not a doctor," she went on. "You don't need to spend all your waking hours worrying about that. Enjoy life. It's okay. We're not trying to ignore the fact that you have those issues in your life, but to absorb yourself in them isn't right either. That's all you talk about."

She was really right. I was always talking either about the next doctor's appointment or the last one, or the next study or the next blood draw or the last one, or some new study I'd read about that they were doing in LA or new medicines, or that bleed that I had in '66, or whatever it happened to be.

"Isn't there more to you than that?" she asked.

We're still together.

Knowing that someone is interested in me in spite of all my medical issues has brought me a new level of confidence and independence. It has probably given me more independence even from my own folks, because I did a lot with them. They were my social life, you know. We'd go to plays and concerts together all the time. I did a lot of stuff with my folks. Now, I have a whole new life, which I never had before. It's nice going out to dinner with somebody other than my parents because when you're in your forties and you're still just going out with your mother and father for dinner, or when you're always traveling with your folks, it's sort of strange.

Love was always something that was missing in my life. I sort of accepted the fact that I should just plain be happy still being on this earth, and if love never happened in my life, well, so be it. It just wasn't meant to be, and I should just be humbly happy that I'm not six feet under, like several other people I knew.

I guess that now I probably would look for empathy rather than sympathy in health care providers. It's okay to be empathetic, to appreciate the situation for what it is, but to say, "Oh, I'm real sorry that you had to go through all this," and "Oh, that's really unfortunate," and, "Oh, poor you," and all this kind of thing, isn't always good. That kind of sympathy isn't always endearing from a health care professional. Don't encourage the "woe is me" kind of attitude about things, or, as my lady friend says, "Buck up."

To parents who find out that their child has hemophilia, I would still say the same thing about becoming absorbed and active. Network with other people. Maybe realize and appreciate some of the toils that people like myself or my folks went through trying to get funding, trying to make a difference, trying to make it a little easier both for ourselves and also for the generations of today who are having kids. We were test dummies without necessarily knowing what was going on.

Look back and appreciate that, too.

It's nice to think that there are some compassionate people out there who are active in the hemophilia industry and who help promote the efforts of people with HIV and hep C. I remember when we were trying to get the *Ricky Ray Bill* passed, my U.S. Senator held it up. It was sitting on his desk. He wouldn't sign it and he wouldn't let it go through the Senate. It had all the required signatures, but it had to go over his desk because he was the liaison to the Department of Health. It sat on his desk because he wouldn't fund it until it included all the other people, other than hemophiliacs, who had been infected with HIV through random blood transfusion. I was getting calls from people in national organizations hoping I could put some kind of pressure on the U.S. Senator from Vermont.

I went down to his office, but he was called into an important meeting and didn't make our meeting. I didn't help that bill along at all, but we held a protest outside the Senator's Vermont office. I'm not sure if he was there that day or not, but he didn't come out if he was. Several moms of young kids with hemophilia came and that was nice. This was long after they had heat-treated the product, but the fact that those moms and dads showed up, it was like, "Hey, yeah, we're in this together," and they all said the same thing.

"You know, today it's HIV. Who knows what else is lurking in the blood that could come back to haunt us? We need to stay together as a community."

There's so much that you want to forget and there's so much that you want to remember, so what do you remember and what do you cast to one side?

Theodore Frost

THEODORE FROST

Mr. Theodore Frost was born in Haverhill, Massachusetts in 1915. Theodore, who is married and has no children, works as a carpenter. He has many memories of years spent in the hospital when he was a child and the miracle of factor VIII when it arrived. He has mild factor VIII deficiency.

They found out my kid brother was a bleeder when he had his tonsils out. He lived until he was seven years old, when he fell out of the car and landed on his head on the granite curb. That took him. That was back in 1927, or very close.

My mother had a nervous breakdown when my brother died.

When I was five and a half years old, I was dragged on the back of a truck, with my feet up on the tailboard chain, out across the old car tracks, which they left sticking up. The streetcars used to go by the house and I was dragging out across the railroad tracks, bump, bumpety, bump, bump, bump. I got a double fractured skull.

It was a case of having to operate. That one accident kept me in the hospital for almost three years. I have a bumpy head from that time.

All of us boys were carpenters. I played around with circular saws and I played around with lathes; I put roofs, new foundations and sills on houses. Whatever was needed, anything pertaining to construction, I did it.

When you got to bleeding internally and started to swell, you suffered and, well, you just handled it. That's all. You did the best you could. As they say "Don't talk about it, do it." I don't complain. I'm still alive.

I went down to report for service around 1940 and they said, "Go home. Stay alive." With the hemophilia, they didn't want me to clutter up the landscape.

When I was a little fellow, and I say *little fellow*, my parents bought me a football helmet and I wore that for a while for protection. I put the football helmet to one side, more for the reason that you'd be walking along and all of a sudden, bang, somebody's hit you on the head.

"Does that hurt? Does that hurt?"

So you're wearing a football helmet to protect you and they've got to see whether it hurts or not when you're hit.

If I saw any rough stuff going on, then I just quietly walked away.

We didn't have any children. My wife had a goiter when she was younger, for which she had an operation, and I had so many x-rays and stuff like that, we figured it was just as well not to have any children. With the hemophilia and me and, well, we never had any kids, anyway.

I'm a factor VIII. They labeled me as minor. Thank God it was just minor. Thank God they didn't throw the whole barrel at me.

I've tried to pinpoint as near as I can when I first received factor VIII. I was bleeding because I had kidney stones and I began to bleed internally. I was up at the Old Hale and I was bleeding in my urinary tract.

"Well, Ted," the doctor said, "you've been bleeding two weeks, and we're not getting anywhere."

"They have a new medicine," he said, "that they want to try on a human being." That was factor VIII, and they classed me as a human being.

Do you want to sign a release, sign your life away, so that they can try that, or not?

It was up to me. I could sign my life away and try it or I could lie there and bleed to death. They called California and told them to ship the factor, which I consented to try. It came by airplane to Boston and the Haverhill Police Department went in and got it. The doctors and nurses gave it to me, which was a show job. In other words, it was new.

That was the beginning of it and they gave me a transfusion of factor. Sealed me right up, just like that. Then there was quite awhile there that if I had internal bleeding or a bad bruise or anything, that's what they would give me, factor VIII. It kept me alive and changed the taking care of me entirely because they didn't even put me in the hospital.

There's so much that you want to forget and there's so much that you want to remember, so what do you remember and what do you cast to one side?

Theodore died in February, 2006

My dad and I were like best friends. We always did things together — building and painting, and we went out in a boat because I grew up on the Vineyard. We were on the boat every weekend. We went fishing, clamming, quahoging, all kinds of neat stuff.

He was always there and we spent a lot of time together. It helped me a lot. It helped me develop into who I am today.

Stephen Place

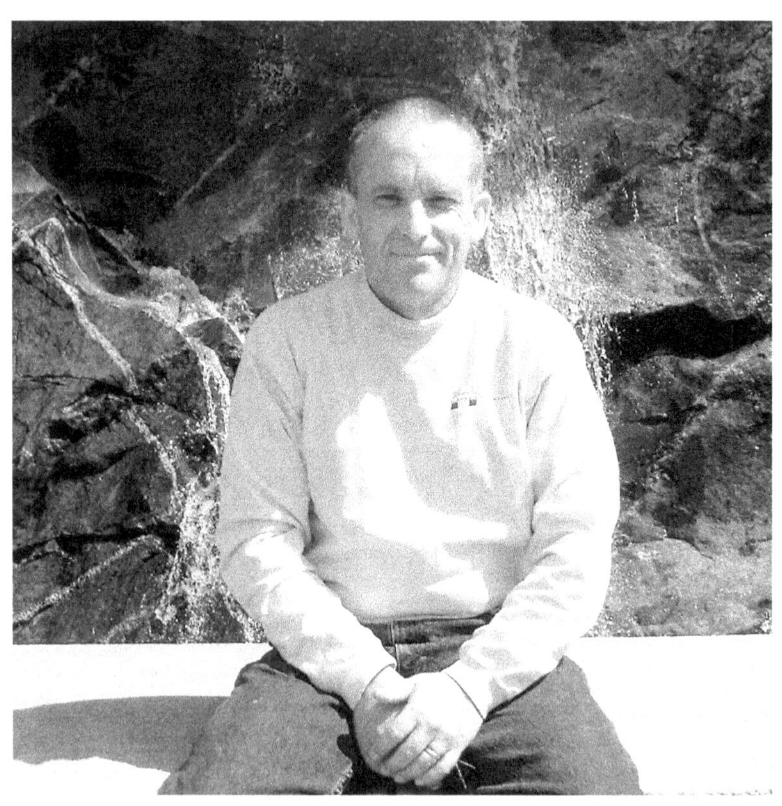

Stephen at Lake Willoughby in Vermont, close to Burke Mountain.

STEPHEN PLACE

Mr. Stephen Place was born in 1954 in Oak Bluffs on Martha's Vineyard. Stephen, who has worked in sales, is married and has two daughters. He has a nephew with hemophilia. He believes you must "know your limits and go to the limit." He has mild factor VIII deficiency.

My mom's brother actually died of a tonsillectomy when he was twelve. That would probably have been in the late '20s, early '30s, when he died. I'm certain that he died of hemophilia; he bled to death.

When I was eleven I fell off my bike riding no-handed. To this day I do not take my hands off those handlebars.

After the bike accident, I had a huge lump on my head. It was almost as big as an egg and it was right smack in the middle of my forehead. A doctor came to the house and said, "Yup, he's got a lump on his head. Just put a compression bandage on it." They didn't know about aspirin being an anticoagulant then. So his head hurts, okay, give him some aspirin. But I'm here, I survived.

After the trauma of the bike accident, I knew that I had hemophilia and that I could get hurt. I remember making a firm decision that I was going to respect my hemophilia, but I was not going to be afraid of it. I was not going to allow anybody to make choices for me, as much as you can as an eleven or twelve-year-old person. I was going to be making choices about what I wanted to do, how far I wanted to venture.

Dr. Ganz was at Mass General and he was pretty important, pretty high up at MGH. He had a summer home on Martha's Vineyard, which is how we got to know him. He was one of these old, stern-type doctors, but a nice guy, and he would say "Well, I don't want you doing this," or, "I don't want you doing that," and I'd go home and probably do it anyway.

I can remember deciding, "I'm not going to let this make me into a whuss."

I know my limits and I'm going to go to those limits. If I cross the line, I could get hurt and I'll pay the price.

Moms and dads worry at different levels: moms are always worried about their children. My dad would say, "Don't worry about it. Don't think about it a lot."

As a young child, I think my dad was the one who was more apt to let me make a choice.

"Well, that's not really good for him, you know," Mom would say. "We have to worry about the hemophilia," da da ... da da ... da da.

My dad bought me a Swiss army knife and the first thing he did when he came home was he went down into the cellar, took this brand new knife and dulled it on a whetstone. He just dulled it right down to almost nothing. So the first thing I did, I opened it up and said, "Oh, it's so sharp!"

My dad would say, "Let him live. Let him have a good life. Let him enjoy himself. Don't coddle him."

I think it caused conflict with my sister because I was the special one. The baby is always the special one, but I had hemophilia, so the extra precautions or maybe the extra trips to Boston bothered her. Kids are very protective of their territory and their rights and the "it's not fair" kind of thing.

When you have something like hemophilia, you don't know what it's like not to have hemophilia. If you bang yourself, you're going to get a bruise. Okay, you've got a bruise. So you have it for five days and someone else has it for two days. Just a way of life.

I waited a couple of years and then finally I decided to get a test. I got the test and then I waited. Well, the doctor was out of the office for the whole week, so I had this terrible week. It was horrible just waiting, but he said, "You're clean and you're clear." Of course, they didn't know about hep C then, either.

My wife and I talked about having kids. We knew that my daughters could be carriers and that their sons would have a fifty-fifty chance of having hemophilia. Also, we knew from all the doctors we've spoken to that their disease would never be more severe than mine. We decided to go ahead.

We know now that there are factor products that take care of it very quickly.

If I am doing something, I look at a couple of important points: head, knees, elbows. If I bump or bang something, you know, a fairly good rap, I'll run right up and get some of my Stimate. Shhh, Shhh, a couple of squirts, put it back in the fridge and I'm right back outdoors doing whatever I was doing.

Don't be afraid that you can't do something because there are a lot of things that you *can* do, especially now with the factor. Now, people with serious hemophilia can probably do more than I can.

Sometimes I wish I didn't have hemophilia, especially when I'm sitting down in a chair for a week with a bad knee. But now, since the factor is pure, if I did really mess up my knee, I'd get some factor into me. I would leave that line in there and then instead of being a week sitting down, it would be a couple of days.

So it does make the quality of life much better, knowing that the factor is there.

I'm a Born-Again Christian. I always thought I had a good relationship with God, but this relationship with Jesus is much better. It really is. From then on, I just kind of dedicated my life to doing whatever I can to serve Him.

I also know that there are going to be tough times. Just because you're Born Again doesn't mean that life's a bowl of cherries.

I can go to God and say, "Help me through this time," and He always has. Every time. There's never been a time that God's let me down. Never.

Honestly, God made me this way, so I'm going to take what He's given me and make the absolute best I possibly can out of it.

Most of the patients I met did not want to be ruled by, or defined by, their disease, but to find, instead, a way to live with it as best they could.

They did not want their hemophilia to run the show.

Cathy Cornell

CATHY CORNELL

Cathy Cornell, LICSW, served as Executive Director of the New England Hemophilia Association from 1995-2006. Before that, she worked as the social worker for the Boston Hemophilia Center at Children's Hospital and at Brigham and Women's Hospital, caring for patients with bleeding disorders and their families. She has more than 25 years of experience as a clinical social worker in medical and mental health settings.

When I completed my degree in social work, I started to look for jobs and I answered an ad for a position in a chronic illness clinic at Children's Hospital. When I arrived for the interview, I learned that it was a social work position in the hemophilia clinic. That was how I started. Hemophilia was a new field for me.

What was really new for me and quite wonderful was working as part of a multi-disciplinary team, with nurses, doctors and physical therapists. I really enjoyed that, and I had the good fortune to have a medical director who valued social work and understood the benefits that social work could offer. I was learning so much.

I had a lot to learn about living with a chronic illness. Most of the patients I met had the attitude that you deal with what's given you; you cope with what you have because you have to. They did not want to be ruled by, or defined by, their disease, but to find, instead, a way to live with it as best they could. They did not want their hemophilia to run the show. That was really inspiring!

When I started at Children's Hospital in Boston in 1988, it was the beginning of the very painful times for the hemophilia community. In fact, the first day I went to work, I got word of a young patient who had died of AIDS. The nurse, who had been working with that patient, was really distressed. Along with many other people, I think she was recognizing that AIDS was going to be taking a big toll on people with hemophilia.

I think that in the beginning there was a kind of hope against hope that maybe HIV was not going to develop the same way in the hemophilia

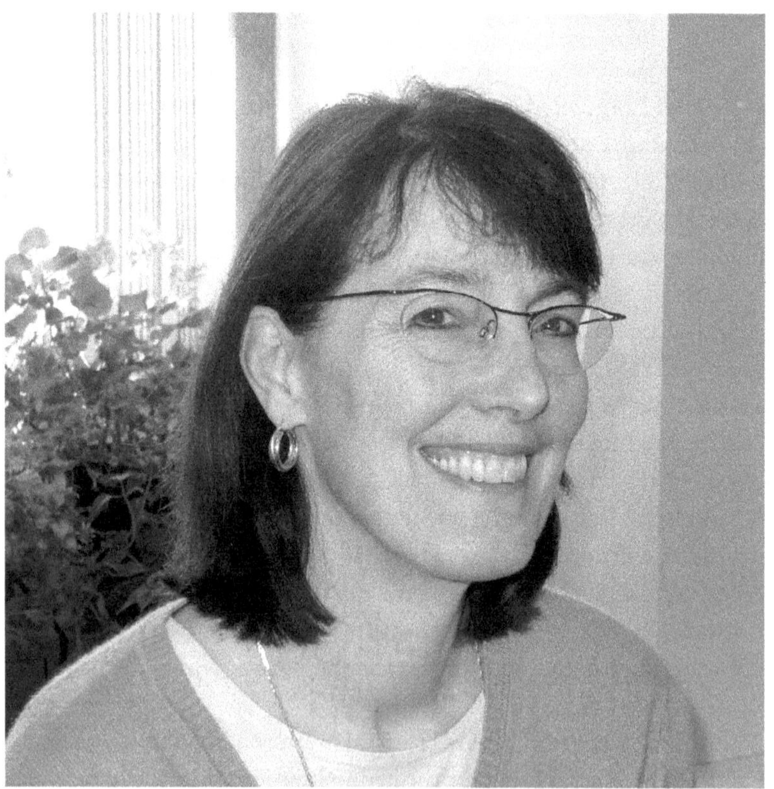

Cathy Cornell

population as it was developing in the gay population, but that hope was a very thin thread. I remember going to a conference and hearing a doctor from Canada really disabuse people of that notion. There was some thought that because the hemophiliacs' immune systems had been bombarded with blood products, maybe they had developed some special resistance, but as time went on that was obviously not to be the case.

It was terrible. In trying to impart hope and perspective to patients, I remember saying things like, "This disease has a long incubation period," "There's promising research," "It's not an immediate death sentence," but it was very, very difficult to find hopeful viewpoints and comforting words.

I vividly remember the shock and despair of one fifteen-year-old on being told that he was positive, and the striking reaction of another boy of twelve or thirteen who, when his mother told him that he had HIV, said simply, "What about my kids?" He instantly fast-forwarded to how this would affect his children and his vision of the future.

Wow, where did that come from? Who would expect a thirteen-year-old boy to be thinking about his future children?

There was a tremendous amount of shock and then some denial. Some people rationalized that being HIV positive meant that you had been exposed, but it didn't necessarily mean that you had, or would have, the disorder. There was confusion about that. And, in fact, there have been some long-term survivors – the non-progressers.

For parents, there was the excruciating issue about when and how you tell your child.

There was a lot of fear about being identified with the gay and drug-user communities; it was about the stigma attached to HIV. Today, we sometimes forget how stigmatizing HIV was, but in the 1980s and early '90s, there were tremendous and irrational fears about HIV, fears which led to discrimination and even violence. There still is anxiety, but nothing like it was then. The whole issue of "to disclose or not to disclose" was huge. Whom do you tell in the family? Do you tell your child's school? Dentist? etc. etc. Some families were open while others lived with a closely-held secret.

We needed to respect the fact that people were all over the map about what they were comfortable disclosing. On occasion, it raised ethical questions, such as when an HIV positive patient did not share the fact with his wife. There were sometimes very difficult situations in the hospital, where parents refused to tell their adolescent kids about their diagnosis. Whose is the right to know? The dilemma for the treatment team was how to talk to the patient about the treatment, but also respect the family's wishes.

There was some feeling among the more outspoken activists that you actually harmed the hemophilia community by staying silent. Many people with hemophilia did speak out courageously for justice and for their treatment needs.

There's a child and his mother who really stay in my mind. He was eight or nine, and his mother had a very, very difficult time hearing what it meant that her son was HIV positive, that this could be related to AIDS and that maybe he should be taking some medication for that. I do remember the point at which she understood, and on one of her visits to the hospital, her attitude seemed different. She had stopped resisting and she allowed treatment to begin. While that was a good thing, it was very painful for her.

That boy fought AIDS for years. Finally, when he was very sick, I remember he said to her, "Mom, I'm so tired." It was then that his mother was able to let him go and that's when he died.

I went through several years with that family and through his death in the hospital. At the funeral, I learned that the mother had lost another child earlier, a daughter, information she had never shared with us.

Through that experience, I realized how little I knew. I thought that I was quite close and involved with the mother and her son, and I was, but I didn't know a huge piece of information about their experience. It is simply intolerable sometimes for people to talk about things that are so painful.

Times are different in hemophilia now. There are new families whose kids are not at risk with HIV. There is prophylactic treatment. There are kids who are playing sports. Even a few years ago, sports would have been out of the question for them. But there's also a gap, this loss, of a whole generation of people and I'm very aware of that and the community is, too. When we try to organize programs, you suddenly think, gee, who is there to mentor these younger kids or talk to the parents?

There are so few people who are still with us.

One fellow told me that he grew up thinking he would be dead by his early twenties. Then factor concentrate was developed and he was given a new lease on life. He began to realize that he could live a long life.

Then he got AIDS and he saw his life expectancy shrink down again.

People with expensive chronic illnesses have a lot to worry about right now with maintaining their insurance and being able to afford or find insurance programs. I know one particular young adult in his twenties who doesn't want to be on disability, but his job doesn't offer him a policy that will cover factor. As companies cut back their plans — and now we're getting these catastrophic or low-cost plans — it's a very serious situation. That issue is very much on our agenda here. We now have a very active advocacy committee that is trying to pass legislation here in Massachusetts to protect access to care.

When I left the hemophilia clinic at Children's, I was up to here with grief. I felt as though I just couldn't bear any more.

I came to understand a lot about the doctor-patient relationship. Interacting with doctors and, more broadly, managing the medical system, is a whole separate field in which people with chronic illness become very expert. Doctors who care for patients over a period of years almost become members of the family.

Every parent of a child with hemophilia will tell you that you must learn to be an advocate for your child. Sometimes you have to be able to contradict what a doctor tells you if you think he's telling you the wrong thing. With a rare disorder like hemophilia, you will have doctors who don't know about hemophilia. They ask some hysterical questions: "How did you get hemophilia?" or "How long have you had it?" That's a tip off.

People with hemophilia use the Internet much more now. The most wonderful thing that I know of on the Internet is a group of "hemo-mommies," as they call themselves. They all have kids with hemophilia and keep in touch through an email group. One of the parents recently had a baby who came down with childhood leukemia, and this group of moms has been taking meals to her. People come down from New Hampshire because it's their turn to take a meal to this family or visit them in the hospital. These people are really standing by one another.

But the Internet can cut both ways. It has also happened that people start giving inappropriate medical advice, which becomes confusing or even damaging.

For this reason, we have decided, as an organization, that we're not going to sponsor chat rooms. We would have to monitor them and we don't have the ability to do that.

Some of the parents of today's children lived through the bad times because they had fathers or brothers or uncles with hemophilia, and I think if they have a family history, they certainly know what has changed.

Others don't really understand the history, and one of our jobs at NEHA [New England Hemophilia Association] is to let those parents know what happened. We need to help them appreciate the contributions made by the people who fought so hard for recognition and compensation, so that this will never happen again.

The hardest part, I find, is trying to explain to young people today what I went through — from having nothing by way of treatment, to where they are today. It's me saying, "You don't know how hard it was when I was a kid growing up," but they don't want to hear that stuff.

Matty Vieira

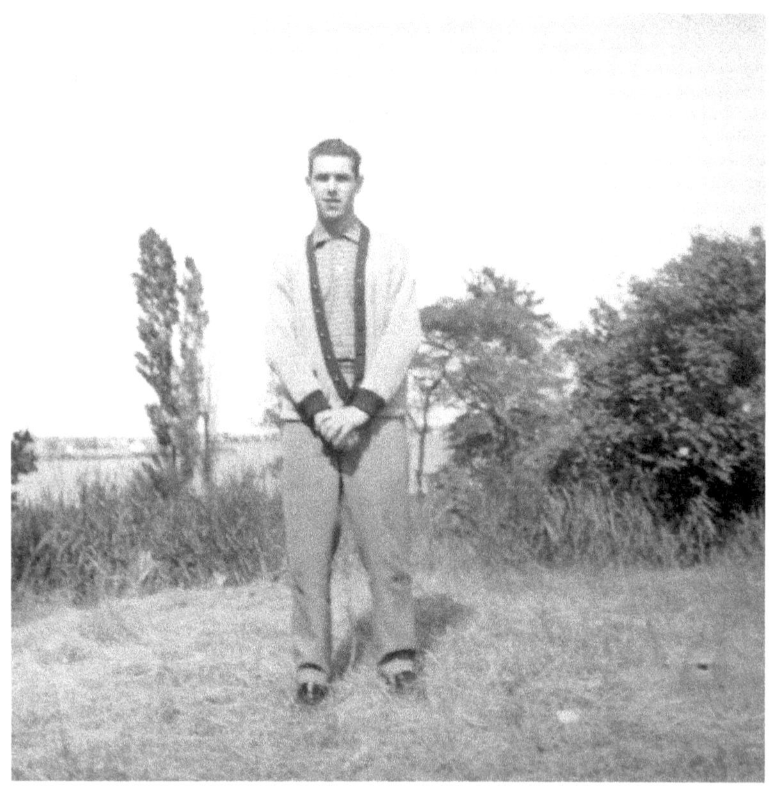

Matty, age 25, in 1959.

MATTY VIEIRA

Mr. Matthew Vieira was born in 1934 in East Boston, Massachusetts. His father, who was Portuguese, worked as a truck driver. Matty had two sisters and describes his home as "Just an average American family."

Mr. Vieira has two sons and one daughter. He and his wife, Eleanor, are very involved with the hemophilia community and feel that support is critical in coping with the disease. Matty was diagnosed with severe factor VIII deficiency at age six. He was successfully treated for his hepatitis C.

Basically, my life changed when I was diagnosed with hemophilia in that I had to be very careful about whatever I did. Of course, my mother and father were very cautious about me not doing anything. Other than that, I tried to lead a normal life. We didn't disclose my condition to anybody because at that time they used to call hemophiliacs "bleeders." Even my teachers didn't know.

Hemophilia — I don't know if people even knew what it was then. They'd say a "bleeder," and people thought that when you got a cut you'd bleed all over them, so it wasn't too public then. I tried to keep it under the table.

My first experiences were at the City Hospital in Boston, and it was for cuts and stuff that I had, and extraction of teeth. Most resident doctors knew nothing about the disease, but it was as good as they could do then. When they came in to see me, they would look at me and I don't know if they expected to see a basket case or what, but they'd look at the chart once and they'd say, "This is Matthew," and I know what they were looking at, you know.

I mean, they knew nothing about hemophilia. They would ask me the same questions over and over again, like "Who had it? When did you know you had it?" The questions were sometimes a pain in the neck, but I knew why they were asking, because none of them knew anything about it. The care was the best they had. Later, we moved on to New England Medical Center with Peter Levine in Boston.

Naturally, I was a little worried about HIV, but I wasn't too concerned because I was one of those people who never infused, probably when I should have. That's why I have a bad knee and a bad ankle from constant bleeds, and it's killed the cartilage.

If I was to come back in life, my next life, I'd know enough to infuse. That was one of the things they always used to tell me, "When in doubt, infuse," which I never did. They were saying, if you've got a little pain or a twinge, infuse.

Even in the early stages, they said always infuse because it's not going to hurt. You can infuse all you want and it won't harm you. It's just going to go in and make your blood healthier, so infuse. I never got to that point. Part of the problem was that in order to get a transfusion, I had, literally, to go to the hospital. I was always thinking that I was going to use up my insurance cap, which I could never have used up in a million years. I would never have gone over my cap at the time. I never will now.

So, not being infused had to do with insurance and it had to do with going back and forth to the hospital.

The cryoprecipitates were a step up, but the best thing that happened in the whole thing was factor VIII and self-infusion. Suddenly, there was the idea that we could have operations if we needed them, with no problems. Factor was a great, great thing for everybody because you could infuse yourself. That was the biggest innovation. You no longer had to go to a medical center or a hospital. You'd call them up and tell them you had a bleed and they'd tell you to infuse. We have our needles and syringes and my wife would infuse me or I'd infuse myself. Now I infuse myself and maybe take it easy for a day or so, and keep in touch with them. You didn't have to keep running back and forth to the hospital the way you did before.

There was one time when Dr. Levine called and said that they had received a notice that there was a bad batch of factor VIII. Fortunately, I didn't have that batch, so there was no problem. Other than that, I never really thought about it.

I said to myself, "Well, I feel awful bad for everybody who has HIV, but it's not my problem. It's not me."

That probably wasn't right, but I think it's like a lot of things. Even today, you find that nobody gets too involved with anything until it affects them personally.

I went to Newman Preparatory School in Boston for about six months after I graduated from high school, then, for some reason, I just left and went to work. I think most of my early jobs were in clerical work or shipping and receiving, stuff like that. Eventually I got into truck driving, and I drove a truck for forty or forty-five years.

I remember one time someone said, "Don't say you have hemophilia, just say you have a factor VIII deficiency." That sounds a little better. It means the same thing, but when you tell someone about the deficiency, it kind of stumps them and they don't ask any more questions. They don't really know what it is, I don't think, but it suffices.

If you say, "I have hemophilia," which is a factor VIII or factor IX deficiency, all kinds of bells and whistles go off and they start asking questions.

I don't think it will ever happen in my time, but they're talking about gene therapy and the possibility that some day, hemophilia may not be there. It will be one of the diseases people "used to have." They'll say, "Well, you know, forget about it," because they've cured it, and then another disease will come along.

The hardest part, I find, is trying to explain to young people today what I went through — from having nothing to treat with — to where they are today. It's me saying, "You don't know how hard it was when I was a kid growing up," and they don't want to hear that stuff.

I say, "You guys are so lucky."

I think people still resent the fact that they have the disease, but it's a lot easier to handle today than it was when I was a kid. I try to help them as much as I can.

The only surgery I had as a child was the extraction of teeth and that was a holocaust. Back then, they would only take a couple of teeth at a time because of the difficulties. They would put you in the hospital and give you pints of whole blood, then they would do the surgery with the one or two teeth and pack it with what they called an oxycell, which was supposed to be some kind of a coagulant.

Then they would take an impression of your teeth, almost like what

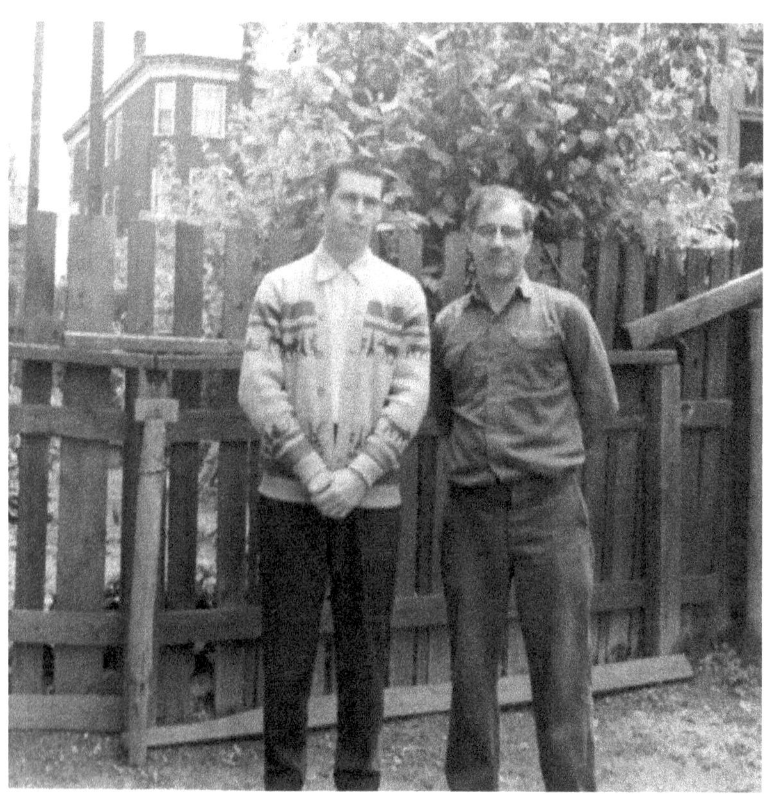

Matty at age 26, with his father, 1960.

people wear today as a mouthpiece, close your mouth and wrap your head with gauze bandages so that you couldn't open your jaws. I had only liquids for about two weeks or so. You weren't supposed to move your mouth at all and I had to stay in bed. There was a lousy taste in your mouth.

Eventually it would heal, over a couple of weeks or so. It was a terrible process, but it was all they knew.

Today it's a lot different. I went to the dentist and had a tooth out a couple of years ago and I infused with my factor. I also had gum surgery. There were no bandages, no oxycell, no nothing like that. I just came home and went back to work the next day.

It's come a long way. It's almost like anyone else having a tooth out.

They were trying to cure people who had hepatitis C with interferon. Mine was peg interferon, which is used for leukemia: same medicine, but it works in different ways. They sent me to see Dr. Grace and he told me that there was a possibility they could cure the hep C. There was no guarantee of anything. He told me that there are a lot of side effects from the drug. Basically, it zaps all your strength; you lose your appetite; you lose weight.

My biggest problem was that I lost weight, about thirty-five to forty pounds. My appetite was suppressed. I didn't feel like eating. I was very tired. I'd come up a flight of stairs from the basement and I'd be huffing and puffing. A couple of times I felt like I had the flu or something.

Here I was, about sixty-eight at the time, and I was saying to them, "Why do you want to put me on this? I'm probably going to die in ten years or so anyway."

"Well," they said, "that's not the way to look at it."

"You might live to be a hundred if we can cure this."

I've been off the interferon now for a year and a half to two years and they can't find any signs of the virus. I've had my blood checked, and they still can't find it. I don't feel as tired and I put some weight back on. So in my case it worked out well for me.

Maybe I will live to be a hundred.

I would say to kids who are born with hemophilia today that the key is to have as normal a life as possible. Even though I'm sure parents would be concerned about the idea of having their kid playing soccer or playing baseball, they should encourage them to do everything that every other kid is doing.

Dr. Will Somers

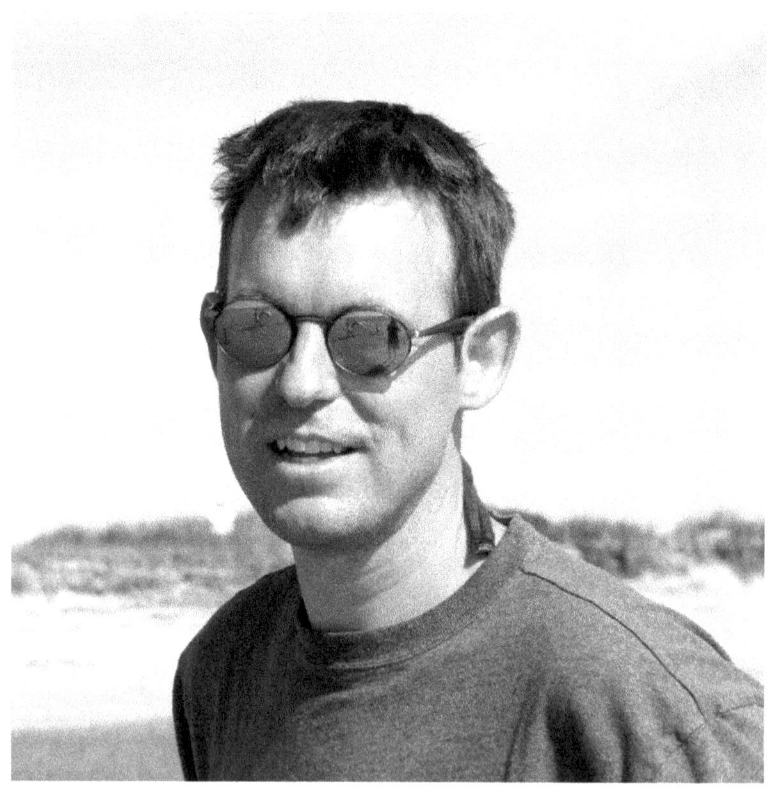

Will Somers

DR. WILL SOMERS

Dr. Will Somers was born in 1964. He grew up and attended university in England, earning a Ph.D. in biophysics. He is married, has a son and currently resides and works in the United States. Will believes that being physically fit is key to counteracting the negative effects of his disease. Dr. Somers has mild to moderate factor VIII deficiency and hepatitis C.

If I really hit my leg or something, I'd be thinking, "Oh, God, now I've got to go to the hospital." I wouldn't go home instantly. I'd get home in the evening and I'd be like, "Okay, I did this, we're probably going to have to do something about it." It was not something that was enjoyable. You have to come to terms with the fact that you're going to have to go the hospital and get the shot and perhaps be limping around for a couple of weeks.

There was one time when I hurt my hip and it was sort of an odd situation. For some reason, I didn't treat it for a few days or a week. I remember being in the hospital and really hurting; eventually, I started treating it and I got better. I remember that was a long event, maybe three or four weeks. I remember on that occasion I was in a children's ward. I got into trouble with the nurses because we put talcum powder on the beds, then bashed them and made all this smoke. I must have been pretty young.

I never really had any serious injury from any sport-related activities. Usually, I'd walk into the corner of a table or something, and that would cause an injury. In part, the way to deal with this is to get fit and be as active as you can. I don't think anyone ever told me that; it was just something I did. I was always running around doing things, and I certainly noticed that the fitter I was, the less trouble I had.

When I went to university, it would literally be once a year or once every few years that I had to deal with an injury. It really was very infrequent at that point. Gradually, injuries occurred less and less as I got older. I wasn't being thrown over my brother's shoulder anymore. I really think a lot of it has to do with how fit you are, and at university I was lifting weights and swimming and windsurfing and scuba diving and doing all this kind of stuff. I was in pretty good shape back then.

I tell you, the worst thing that happened was when I was at university. I had a bleed into my stomach area and that went on for a couple of months. I didn't really know what the problem was. I was feeling dizzy, I knew I had lost some blood and I could see I was pale, but I had no money. I walked to the pharmacy and I was going to get some iron tablets; the price of the iron tablets was what made me go to the hospital. When I got there they were like, "Okay, don't move. We're going to get an ambulance." They gave me blood. That was probably the most serious thing I ever had, and I actually ended up missing several months of the school year. The situation eventually resolved itself, but it took a long time.

Most of the time, my hemophilia wasn't really an issue for me. I guess when you're lying there and you've got a sore ankle or whatever, you'd rather not be ill. But if you have something that affects you once every couple of years, it really becomes less of an issue.

In the early days, you were getting a very large volume of plasma, and it would take a long time to put it into you. I remember that. I remember lying on the bed just waiting for it to happen. I certainly remember the time I went in and they had these giant syringes instead of the bags. That was a big step forward. It was much quicker, much more efficient. You'd go in and you'd be out of there very quickly.

There was a senior guy in England, Dr. Ritzer, who seemed to be very knowledgeable. He was one of the doctors people looked up to. He seemed to understand what was going on and the nurses were very nice.

It was very different when I came to the hospital here. The first time I visited a hospital in the States at UCSF, I remember standing in a corridor. They were giving me a shot and there were people who seemed to be homeless walking around the corridor talking to me while this was going on. In England, they were all very friendly and it seemed like a very pleasant environment in comparison. Here, I was dealing with health insurance and everything else, and it seemed kind of an odd situation. In England, you just go along to any hospital and they take care of you.

Hemophilia was certainly not something I wanted to talk about with most people. I don't think any of my friends ever knew about it. They still don't know about it. If I entered into a relationship with somebody, if it was going somewhere serious, I would tell them. In the normal day-to-day relationships, I don't think there was any need for people to know.

In England, around birthday times, it's pretty tough. People will come and pick on you and kick you and all this kind of stuff. I don't remember anybody not doing this to me. They treated me as badly as everybody else. When you're a young kid in England, at the school I was at, you get a thing called the 'bumps.' Fifteen people will gather around you, grab an arm and a leg each and then throw you up in the air and kick you on the way down. Obviously, you don't want to let anybody know it's your birthday, but every year someone found out and then this would happen to me. I don't remember them sparing me in any way, so I can't imagine that people knew.

At some point, I think in my early twenties, it got to the point where I could give myself home treatment and that's when it became much easier. Part of the time at university, I was at home giving myself factor. Certainly the volumes are lower now than they were back then but, you know, essentially it's the same kind of treatment and I guess companies are working to try and make it more convenient. But at that point it became pretty good. I don't know why I still avoid using it, although now I'm better about keeping a reasonable supply sitting there. If anything happens, I just take care of it, usually.

In the UK they had something called the Douglas Bader Scholarship Program for people with disabilities, and somehow I managed to join to get my pilot's license. Many of the people were badly disabled and I felt like a fake going in for it because I felt as though I was perfectly healthy compared to the other people who were there. I learned to fly, but there was a restriction placed on me: I had to have somebody else in the cockpit, which is ridiculous, because I was perfectly healthy as far as I was concerned.

With the sports, I do tend to get bruises, small bruises, and a lot of the time I'm thinking, "Okay, well, I'll wait a couple of days and see what happens." Most things just get better. I didn't feel it was worth dealing with the factor VIII, and I guess that's probably still the case now. I'm probably a little more proactive now if I have a feeling it's going to get worse. I'm more realistic about dealing with it quickly now. I'm more realistic in that rather than hoping it's going to get better and then realizing a few days later it's not, I do something.

When people first hear about hemophilia, I don't think they really know all the implications. When I met my first wife, she'd scuba dive with me. I was teaching her to windsurf, and we were hiking and camping and everything, so it's like "Well, big deal. This isn't really a problem." I've met most people through something like scuba diving. I think people assumed hemophilia was never going to really be an issue for me.

I was following all the headlines that were coming out about HIV. I was in England at that time. I hadn't had any treatment for a few years, so I was thinking, "Well, this is probably a good time not to be getting treatment." At some point, there was a real concern about the supply of factor VIII and that was the time when I had this bad, internal bleed, so I went to the hospital. They said, "Well, you have two choices. We have this National Health Service material that we think is higher quality than the American factor VIII, or you can have the heat-treated American factor VIII, which we think is safe."

It was a little bit scary because at that point there didn't appear to be any real hard data about which option was best. Even the doctor didn't seem completely convinced about which way to go, and this made it worse. Oxford seemed to disagree with the Leeds Center. I started treatment in Leeds in the north of England because that's where the university was, with American heat-treated material. When I got down to Oxford, they said they would prefer to switch me onto the National Health Service factor — I guess it came from a small pool of donors.

I certainly remember going to be tested. They gave you a test every six months back then. I guess they weren't sure how long things would take to show up, so I think every six months or so I would go in for a test. I was following the headlines, and I consider myself pretty fortunate.

I remember going to the hospital thinking, "Oh, my God. This is not a good time to be doing this." So I wasn't happy with the idea of having to get factor VIII at that point, but I had it literally every day for a couple of months because of the bleed that I had going on.

My mother wanted me to go to medical school. In England, you have to make the decision to go to medical school when you're eighteen or nineteen, but I had goofed off too much in school. My grades were good enough, but at that point I'd been offered a course in biophysics, and that seemed interesting, so I decided to do that. When that course finished, I was offered the chance to do a Ph.D., so I did the Ph.D. It turned out to be a pretty good career move at the end of the day, but it was one of these things I sort of drifted into.

I'd been in the north of England attending university for seven years and I really wanted a change. I imagined California as this beautiful place with beautiful beaches, so I applied to schools in California to do a post-doc. I ended up going there for a few years, and after you've been in the States for a few years, it's pretty hard to move back.The money is so much better here. It was very difficult at that point to move back.

Mainly what struck me here was the financial situation. You know how much the factor VIII costs. You go to the hospital and I mean basically the hospitals seemed obsessed with getting your insurance card and all this kind of stuff. When I first arrived, I was like, "What is this system?" When I moved house, my bill went to the wrong place and the first thing the hospital did was trash my credit rating. They sent a collection agency after me for the forty-dollar co-pay, or whatever it was. That was my welcome to the U.S. health care system. For the next five years, I couldn't borrow money to buy a pillowcase, thanks to the bad credit rating. In England, you literally don't deal with any of this. You have no concept what factor VIII costs.

The other thing is, you certainly don't see the doctors much here. I think in England I always viewed the doctors as somebody I knew. I saw Dr. Rizza all the time I was growing up. It seems that people here move around a lot more. It's certainly hard for me to keep track of the people I'm supposed to see at the center here. Basically, you go in and they see you; you get the problem dealt with; you leave. Often for me by the next time I go in, there's a different set of people. I haven't stayed in the hospital in the States since I arrived here. Usually they try and get you out of there as quickly as they can. In England, it doesn't seem to be as big a deal having you stay over.

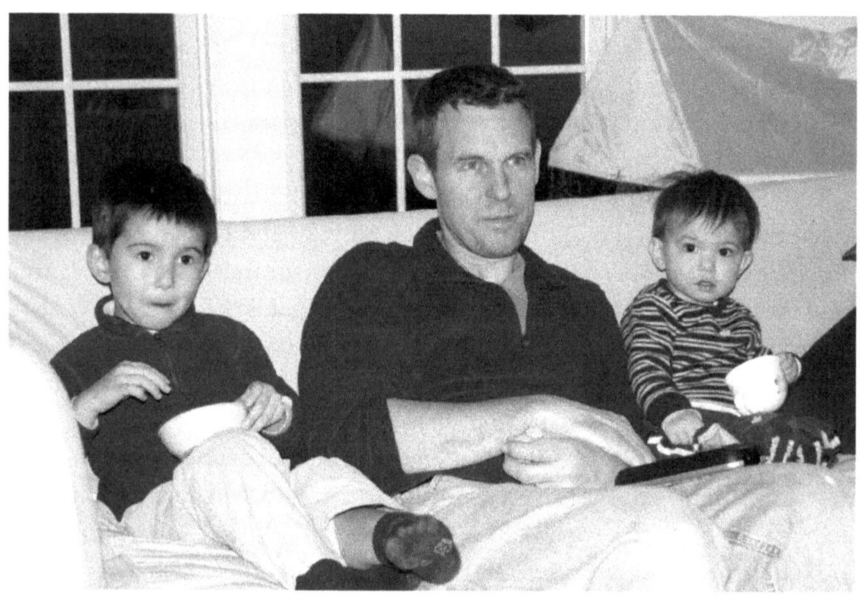

"A typical evening in our house."
Will with his two sons, Liam (age 4) on the left and Owen (15 months) on the right.

I do have hep C and I have started finding out more about it.

I just read the report from the lawyers representing the people who have been affected by hep C. If what they say is even half true, it's pretty shocking what the pharmaceutical companies were doing to maximize their profits, particularly in the States, where they bought blood from prisons and these kinds of things.

Having said that, I work for a pharmaceutical company which is on the other end of some litigation — not this particular litigation — so I have mixed feelings about it. Certainly, if these guys were buying blood from prisoners when they were told not to, then they deserve to compensate people and it's pretty outrageous what they did. But I don't really know enough to know whether the lawyers in this case are telling the truth.

I would say to kids who are born with hemophilia today that the key is to have as normal a life as possible. That means that even though I'm sure parents would be concerned about the idea of having their kid playing soccer or playing baseball, they should encourage them to do everything that every other kid is doing. Try and keep them as active as possible and encourage them to be as physically fit as possible. The other thing I believe in is keeping joints in good condition. If you get any joint bleeds, you should deal with the factor VIII as quickly as possible and move on from there. I have a sore hip now that I think resulted from a hospital stay when I didn't receive treatment for a week or so.

The reality is that the more you protect kids, the more out of shape they'll become and the more bleeds they'll get. I don't think it helps to try and protect people.

The only thing that ever concerned me was one time when I was traveling after I finished university. When I went into a remote part of China or Thailand, I would think, "Okay, I'm perhaps a little more isolated than I might otherwise be. I'm certainly some distance away from reasonable treatment." But that's really the only time I've ever been concerned about it. Certainly not when I'm in any situation here.

These days, it's much easier than when I grew up, and even then it didn't slow me down very much. Really the only thing that I'm dealing with now is a few joint issues, and I think that there's no reason to have to deal with that these days.

My hip hurts now when I walk around on it too much, or when I've been windsurfing or kite boarding or whatever. I come in and my hip will hurt after that. So this relates to keeping joints in good condition. Clearly, there was pain associated with these bleeds when I was younger, but it's just one of the things you sort of forget about.

I certainly don't look back and think about being in pain all the time when I was growing up. I don't really think about the pain, although clearly it hurt at the time.

It's hard to know whether hemophilia was part of this, but I've always been very determined to just go and do things and not let anything get in my way. Certainly I think that that attitude helped me in my career. Some people, with work or university or whatever, let obstacles get in the way. I don't let that happen. I'll always try to find a way to get something done, and ultimately that helps me. I've done fairly well.

I think hemophilia led to my attitude: "I'm not going to let things get in my way."

It was a huge responsibility when you knew there was no right answer. We didn't know, and it wasn't as if someone could go out and quickly do an experiment or a clinical trial and answer the questions. We knew that there were going to be answers that would be forthcoming in five or ten years, but we had to make decisions and recommendations and have a dialogue with our families today. It was very challenging.

Dr. Diana Beardsley

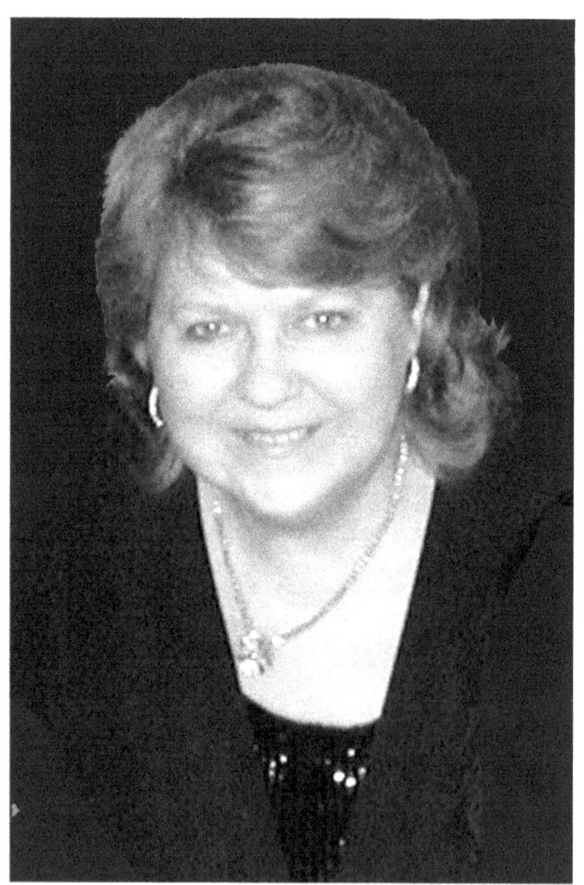

Dr. Diana Beardsley

DR. DIANA BEARDSLEY

Dr. Diana Beardsley, a Wisconsin native, completed her education at Princeton (Ph.D.) and Duke (M.D.) before she moved to Boston to specialize in Pediatric Hematology and Oncology. In 1980, she chose to focus her career on hemophilia and bleeding disorders, thus experiencing the early HIV era first hand. Dr. Beardsley established comprehensive hemophilia treatment centers (HTCs) in Boston, Massachusetts and in New Haven, Connecticut. Currently, she is Associate Professor of Pediatrics and Internal Medicine at Yale University School of Medicine. She has been the Medical Director of the Yale HTC for more than twenty years.

I grew up in central Wisconsin on our family farm, and went to a one-room country school where there were eight grades in one room. It had a wood stove and outhouses when I first started, but the school installed indoor plumbing when I was in second or third grade. It was quite an advance! I graduated from eighth grade with five in my class.

Scholarships allowed me to go off and study science, and I majored in chemistry at Valparaiso. After college, I went to graduate school at Princeton, where I did my Ph.D. in physical chemistry. In that era, there was limited support for women going into professions. One of my chemistry professors in college came right out and said he didn't think that women really should be going off to graduate school. When I was a first-year graduate student, the same kind of opinion was voiced – that perhaps the slots should be saved for men who were really going to continue with the profession.

I decided to do my research in the laboratory of Dr. Walter Kauzmann. He's quite a famous physical chemist – famous for his books on thermodynamics and also for discovering the concept of hydrophobic bonding, which is important in protein structure. I remember him telling me about this marvelous group of enzymes, arrayed in a cascade-like fashion, that controlled blood clotting. One enzyme activated another, that augmented the reaction and that activated another. The whole thing was just marvelously balanced. That was my introduction to those proteins and I thought, "You know, this is quite a wonderful system and perhaps some day we'll understand more about it."

In medical school, I found pediatrics and pediatric problems to be very exciting, and I loved working with the whole family. I did my residency in pediatrics and my fellowship in pediatric hematology and oncology at Children's Hospital in Boston. The section chief was David Nathan. I was interested in blood clotting and platelets. Sam Lux at Children's and Bob Handin at the Brigham were supportive of me and helped me. I became interested in platelet immunology and began to study the targets of anti-platelet antibodies. I continue with that investigative work to this day.

Each fellow had to have some clinical focus, and I wanted my clinical area of interest to be hemophilia. The program had been directed by Orah Platt, and she was willing to take me under her wing and guide me in caring for the hemophilia population. So, I was allowed to become a clinical hemophilia specialist and do research on platelet immunology. This was in '80 or '81, when everything was about to change in the hemophilia field!

I remember 1982 very well. In the summer of that year, there was a report that two patients with hemophilia had been diagnosed with the new disease, AIDS, and no etiology was known. It was the first time this had been reported in individuals with hemophilia and it was a little unsettling. A little later, in 1982, an infant who had received multiple blood transfusions was also diagnosed with AIDS.

At the 1982 American Society of Hematology (ASH) meeting we learned that twelve men with hemophilia had been diagnosed with AIDS, so now the picture was becoming very worrisome for my patient population. Maybe our population was not completely different from the groups at risk for this new disease. I recall the meeting where this was presented because it was standing room only. Everyone was cautiously wondering what this was really going to mean down the road, and of course we knew nothing about the cause of this new disease at that time.

I came back to Boston after the ASH meeting and drafted a letter and shared it with David Nathan. We made a plan to invite all the patients and families of the hemophilia population from our clinic to a meeting. I wanted to share what was out there and to explain that we didn't know what it meant. We didn't know where it was going, but we had concerns. I told them that we would stay on top of things and share any information we had with them.

I told the patients and families that I didn't know what was right to do; that we were open to hearing their ideas; and that one idea we had sort of thrown around as a possibility would be to switch patients who were on factor VIII concentrate back to cryoprecipitate. That way, if there was something that was transfusion-transmitted, there would be fewer donors in the cryoprecipitate than there were in the factor concentrates.

I recall a couple of the older patients who had lived through the cryoprecipitate age voicing the opinion that factor concentrates had made their lives so normal and cryoprecipitate had not given them that. They thought if this was something that was coming from the factor – the treatments – they had probably already been exposed to it. One way or another, they didn't want to go back to a different era.

Home infusion had already been started by the generation before my introduction, so most of the older kids were already on home infusion of concentrates, either factor VIII or the prothrombin complex concentrates – PCC's – for factor IX deficiency. It had been our practice to treat the young children with factor VIII deficiency with cryoprecipitate until they were ready for home infusion. The idea was that as long as they were going to have to come to the emergency department for an infusion anyway, we might as well give them the cryoprecipitate, which is not a pooled product. Factor concentrates weren't started until they were on home infusion.

I thought that this was not a good time to take young children who were currently being treated with cryoprecipitate and convert them to factor, not until we understood better what was going on. Families agreed that this seemed like a small price to pay. It wasn't going backwards for anyone.

The other alteration we made in their therapy, which we announced at the meeting, was that we had decided that any truly elective surgery ought to be postponed until we understood the risks a little better.

In the field at large there were a number of responses. One response was – and people would quote statistics – that the greatest cause of death in patients with hemophilia was bleeding, so we shouldn't stop treating bleeding episodes. That opinion was voiced by a number of people.

Another opinion put forward was that if you don't treat a joint bleed early, you're going to end up with a target joint or synovitis, and it will

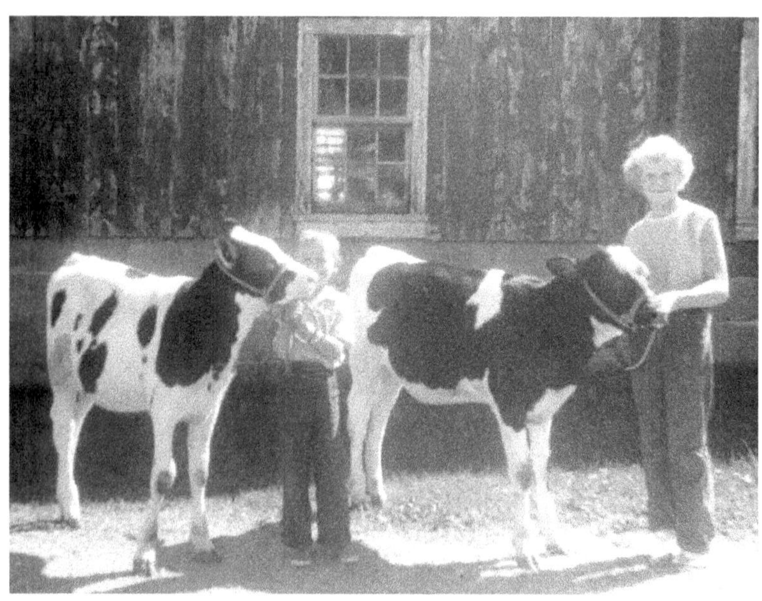

Diana and her brother Brian on the family farm in 1959.

require much more treatment than prompt early treatment would require, so don't stop treating.

I think everyone in the hemophilia community had some uncertainties. We didn't know what the AIDS cases meant. We wondered with only twelve diagnosed individuals whether it could be a coincidence. There were about fifteen thousand men with hemophilia in the country. Did twelve of them just happen to have another risk factor that hadn't yet been uncovered? But within that year it quickly became apparent that blood products were, in fact, a risk factor for AIDS.

In '83 - '84, a heat-treated factor concentrate was developed by Baxter. The initial goal of that therapy was to decrease the risk of hepatitis. The heat-treated factor had been tested in chimpanzees: the chimpanzees that got the heat-treated factor concentrate with the hepatitis B hadn't come down with any disease, whereas all the chimpanzees that received the non heat-treated factor had evidence for hepatitis.

Baxter submitted an abstract for the ASH meeting. However, about a month later, the other chimpanzees also got hepatitis. So the heat treatment didn't completely eliminate hepatitis, but it seemed to delay the onset and maybe modify the severity of the disease.

As soon as the heat-treated factor concentrate became available, I started switching our patients who were on factor concentrate to heat-treated factor concentrate – factor VIII concentrate. I faced some opposition because the heat-treated factor might lose some activity and it cost twice as much as the non heat-treated factor.

Some of my colleagues accused me of generating unnecessary worry and anxiety when we had absolutely no data to support making the switch. That was true; there were no data. There were no studies to prove what was the right thing to do. Some very brilliant people made different choices and didn't make a move that early to heat- treated factor concentrate.

Even after the first HTLV tests were available, we didn't know whether a seropositive result meant that you were almost certainly going to get the disease or whether you were immune to the virus and safe from AIDS. That hypothesis was put forward very legitimately. We just didn't know.

When families heard all this, I think they appreciated our candor. It was a real lesson to me that if you don't know the answer, you can share that.

It wasn't as though you could have a discussion with someone and say, "This is the right thing to do for all of these reasons." It was a matter of judgment. You had to take whatever information – and mostly it was lack of information – that you had at the time and make a recommendation to a patient or a family. I think every clinician in the field made this assessment with the patients' best interests in mind.

It was a huge responsibility when you knew there was no right answer. We didn't know, and it wasn't as if someone could go out and quickly do an experiment or a clinical trial and answer the questions. We knew that there were going to be answers forthcoming in five or ten years, but we had to make decisions and recommendations to our families today. It was very challenging. There was an awful lot at stake, and we had way too little knowledge. I think a lot of what we did was listen, and, more than making firm recommendations, we were having an ongoing dialogue with the families.

Once things had really been spelled out and you could see the extent of the problem, it became really horrifying. People knew friends who were affected or maybe had a brother who had already died of AIDS. That was really awful.

The patients I had who were diagnosed with AIDS were few in number and they were primarily here at Yale – adults and young adults. Because the population at Yale had been switched to heat-treated concentrate fairly early, our HIV exposure rate was well below the national average.

There's not a single death that's easy.

I remember one teenager who came in with a very serious infection. He was known to be HIV positive and he needed massive support in the intensive care unit. The ICU team raised the issue of withdrawing support, since he had a condition that was considered incurable. I remember talking to the intensive care physicians and saying, "You know, we should have a chat with the family because he's not going to be cured of the AIDS, but if he pulls through this infection he would at least have some more life."

The event this teenager was hospitalized for was a bacterial infection that, in fact, he recovered from completely. It was one of his first manifestations of AIDS. He was able to make plans for a number of years of travel and time with his family, and even though there was always the cloud that this was probably not something that was going to be cured and go away, at least he had life given back to him for a period of time.

Part of my hemophilia practice, particularly at Yale, was dealing with young men who were HIV positive who were contemplating marriage and wanting to have children, with all of the unknowns that surrounded that situation. It was really heart-wrenching. There really was no known, completely safe way to have unprotected sex or to have a child. That work was very hard to do.

It was really tragic – tragic for everybody. The one thing I know is that all of us who were caring for patients did what we thought was best for the patients, whether that meant encouraging a more conservative or a more aggressive approach. I think the only motivation was what would be best for the patients. I know there were other people who assessed the situation differently, and all I can say is that at that time, it wasn't clear who was right and who was wrong or what the right approach was.

Hemophilia is an absolutely wonderful area of medicine to be working in. The rate at which advances have been made is astonishing. It usually takes decades for new drugs and improvements in therapy to actually produce clinical benefits, especially for children, but advances have moved with lightning speed in the hemophilia field during my generation. True, the advances have been pushed forward because of the terrible tragedies that occurred – the hepatitis and HIV. Nevertheless, it's been satisfying to see. Families have been a part of the progress – they have been part of the advocacy in a very major way. It's satisfying to know that we're all driving the train in the same direction.

Patients have benefited from heat-treated factor, immunoaffinity purified, recombinant, and now we're looking at longer-acting forms of factor and eventually gene therapy. The whole field thinks in terms of solutions that can actually benefit patients within a reasonable time period.

The comprehensive care model was really developed by my predecessors in the hemophilia field. The founding leaders put it into practice and then documented that it was effective and even cost effective. The comprehensive model applied immediately to HIV care very successfully and we see it in other

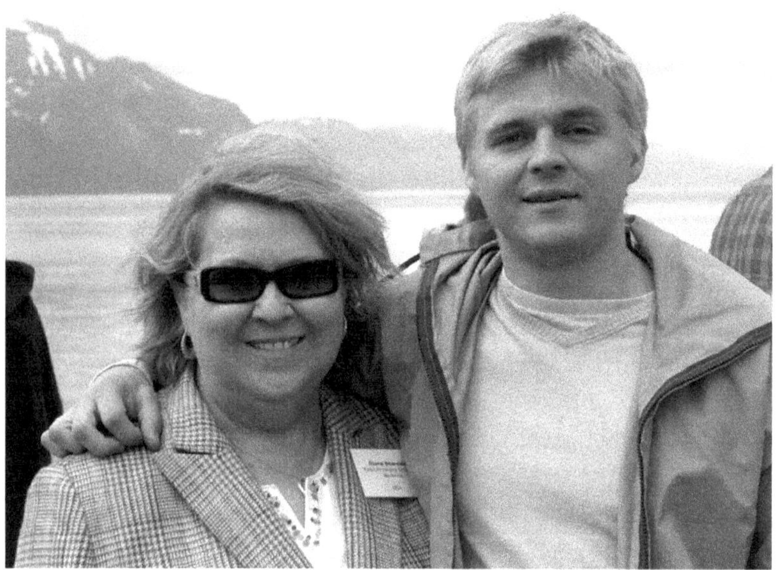

Diana with her son Christopher in 2006.

fields now. I think that hemophilia has probably contributed that collaborative, preventive care type of model to the benefit of many sub-specialties.

In the early 1980s, Bob Handin and I approached the New England Hemophilia Center director and said we really wanted our Boston program to join on and be part of the Regional Comprehensive Center network. Dr. Levine welcomed us very graciously and that was my introduction to comprehensive hemophilia care as it is organized in the United States.

I came to Yale in 1986 and because I'd been director of the Hemophilia Center at Children's in Boston, I worked to get a Hemophilia Treatment Center (HTC) here at Yale. Our center has now been an HTC for more than 20 years.

One thing that's been very satisfying to me, outside the immediate patient care setting in our own center, is the hemophilia community nationally and internationally. Colleagues I've come to know over the years are some of the people I admire most in the world – brilliant people, nice people, very willing to share and available for advice or interaction and collaboration. The academic hemophilia community is one of the real strengths and the reason that I am so grateful that hemophilia became my field of specialty.

We're a tight-knit community and there is a special bond among the hemophilia treaters. Most of us went through an era that was very challenging, and it really brought us closer together.

One of the professionally satisfying things for me, certainly of great benefit to our patients, has been the devotion and dedication of the other members of the hemophilia care team, particularly the nurse coordinators. Comprehensive hemophilia care couldn't exist without the nurse coordinators and the social workers.

When the AIDS risk became apparent I certainly got the impression that manufacturers were moving very quickly. They seemed very anxious to do the right thing in terms of screening their plasma donors by instituting testing as soon as it could be done and then preparing virally safe products. I certainly got the impression that all the actions that were taken did have patient safety right in the foreground.

The hemophilia population has been a wonderful group to work with. I was privileged to get to know many patients and families well enough to share

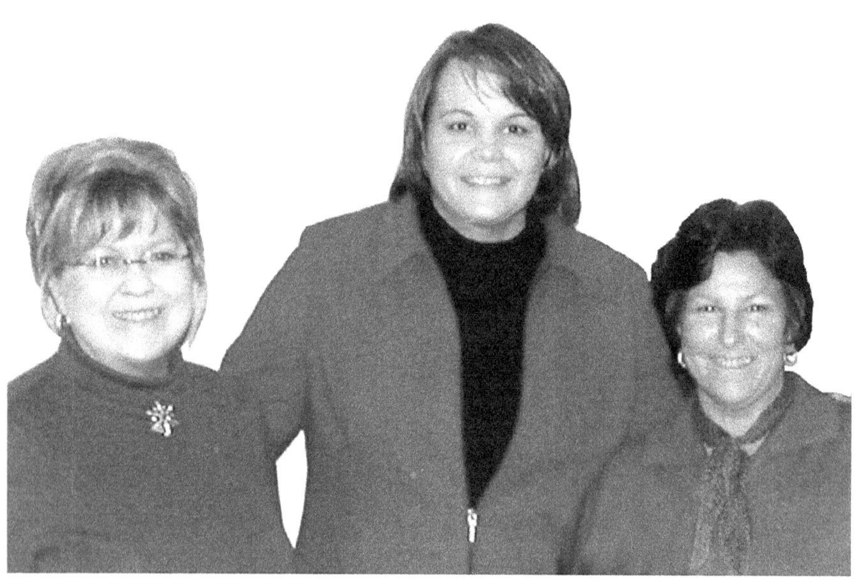

Diana (center) with her Yale Hemophilia Center colleagues, Jennifer Cironi and Susan Marino.

some of the challenges that their disease forced on them as they were growing up or taking on careers. I could see what kind of obstacles they had overcome to succeed in life, and it is a privilege to have known these families over a period of time. One of my young patients was married last year, and I was able to go to his wedding. I mean, this was wonderful. He's a very fine young man.

Today, we encourage parents to expect a normal life for their child with hemophilia. While treatment will be part of that life, it should be in order that the child is not at particular risk. Hemophilia definitely shouldn't limit their ability to do all the important things in life. I'm hoping that we will have a cure for hemophilia. I would like to feel that we could correct factor VIII or factor IX deficiency, if not permanently, at least for a very long period of time. I'm quite confident we will make progress in that direction.

How long it will take remains to be seen.

Glossary*

AIDS (Acquired Immune Deficiency Syndrome) – A disease that attacks and destroys the body's immune system, leaving the patient abnormally vulnerable to infections and many other diseases.

Bleeding disorders – A group of distinct conditions in which a person's body cannot properly develop a clot, causing an increased tendency for bleeding.

Carrier – An individual who possesses the gene for a condition, but does not necessarily have the condition.

Clotting factors – Proteins needed to form blood clots.

Coagulation disorders – A large group of conditions in which a person experiences excessive bleeding or clotting.

Cryoprecipitate – A form of factor VIII-concentrated plasma that was first discovered by Dr. Judith Graham Poole in 1965. While a breakthrough in treatment at that time, it is no longer used as the current standard of treatment in the United States.

Factor deficiencies – These are rare disorders identified by the particular deficient or missing clotting factor in a person's body. These conditions include: Factor I, II, V, VII, VIII, IX, X, XI, XII, and XIII.

Gene – A section of DNA, the chemical code of the body that controls production of a protein.

Gene therapy – A method of replacing, manipulating or supplementing a dysfunctional gene with a functioning one. This evolving technique is currently being researched in several inherited diseases, including hemophilia. There is hope that gene therapy will lead to better treatments, and eventually cures.

Hemoglobin - The protein that carries oxygen and carbon dioxide in red blood cells.

Hematologist – A physician who specializes in disorders of the blood.

Hemophilia – A bleeding disorder in which a specific clotting factor protein, namely factor VIII or IX, is missing or does not function normally.

Hemophilia A – A deficiency or absence of factor VIII. It has also been called "classic" hemophilia.

Hemophilia B – A deficiency or absence of factor IX. It has also been called "Christmas Disease," after the first family that was identified with the condition.

Mild Hemophilia – A categorical term used to describe someone with a factor VIII or IX level ranging from 5% to 40% of normal blood levels.

Moderate Hemophilia – A categorical term used to describe someone with a factor VIII or IX level ranging from 1% to 5% of normal blood levels.

Severe Hemophilia – A categorical term used to describe someone with a factor VIII or IX level below 1% of normal blood levels.

Hemophilia Treatment Centers (HTCs) – A group of federally-funded hospitals that specialize in treating patients with coagulation disorders. Each center has at least a hematologist, a nurse, a social worker, and a physical therapist working as a team to deliver comprehensive care to patients and families.

Hepatitis – A group of viruses that can lead to infection and inflammation of the liver.

Hereditary disease – A condition that is genetically passed down to one's offspring.

HIV (Human Immunodeficiency Virus) – The virus that causes AIDS.

Infusion – A means of delivering treatment to some people with bleeding disorders. This method is used to introduce clotting factor concentrate directly into a vein.

Inheritance – The biological process of transmitting certain characteristics or conditions from parents to offspring.

Orthopedic – A term having to do with the bones, the skeleton or associated structures.

Platelets – These are tiny "plate-like" components of blood that help to seal off injured blood vessels and stop bleeding.

Prophylaxis – A treatment regimen aimed at preventing bleeding episodes among people with hemophilia.

Spontaneous mutation – The development of a hereditary disease for which there is no family history.

Target joint – A term for a particular joint that has experienced repeated bleeds or at least four bleeds into one joint within a six month period.

*Courtesy of the National Hemophilia Foundation, 2007

NOTES

NOTES

NOTES

NOTES

NOTES

NOTES

NOTES

NOTES

www.ingramcontent.com/pod-product-compliance
Lightning Source LLC
Chambersburg PA
CBHW060005210326
41520CB00009B/825

9780980240528